"In a world full of explicit lies, today's kids nee[illegible] afraid to tell them the explicit truth. This book provides parents with the tools they need to have these candid and continual conversations."

—Dr. Kevin Leman, *New York Times* bestselling author
of *Have a Happy Family by Friday*
and *The Birth Order Book*

"Jonathan McKee is one of America's premier youth specialists, and this book will help you navigate the rough waters of teaching your kids healthy sexuality. There are some shocking but true statistics in this book to help you do your job. It's a very good read and can help your kids make good decisions about their sexuality for their lives now and their future."

—Jim Burns, PhD, president, HomeWord
and author of *The Purity Code*
and *How God Makes Babies*

"Parents, take a deep breath. This book pulls no punches. But it will give you exactly what you need to walk alongside your kids at this time when they most need it. Let's become a generation of parents that our children can safely come to for truth!"

—Shaunti Feldhahn, social researcher, speaker,
and bestselling author of *For Women Only*
and *For Parents Only*

"If you're a parent of a teen or several teens like I am, then talking authentically and intentionally about sexuality is a mandatory responsibility in today's world. Failure to do so would be either sheer ignorance or negligence. To this end, Jonathan has written a thorough, straightforward, and engaging resource that will both equip and inform a parent for effective, culturally relevant, and God-honoring conversations about sexuality and all its implications. It is a critical read in critical times."

—Brian Berry, generation ministries pastor,
Journey Community Church, La Mesa, California;
author, *As For Me and My Crazy House*

"SO many parents I know don't feel equipped to talk to their kids about sex. This book helps you overcome the (guaranteed) awkwardness of conversations like that, and provides both tools

AND motivation. I wish every parent would read it . . . their kids would be the ones who'd benefit!"

—Scott Rubin, director of middle school ministry,
Willow Creek Community Church

"We shouldn't just wait for someone or *something* else to help our children navigate the confusion and deception that they experience regarding sex. Jonathan McKee is both a parent and a trusted expert on adolescence and youth-related issues. In this book, he provides clarity and practical knowledge so that you and I can do more than just give a nervous 'talk' to our kids; we can be loving and consistent parents for them as well."

—Terry Linhart, PhD, educator, author,
Bethel College—Indiana

"Kids need parents who are educated, aware, and relevant when it comes to sex. Thankfully, Jonathan McKee gives us powerful, poignant, and practical tools to help us win in this delicate and scary parenting arena. Read this and gain hope and confidence."

—Doug Fields, co-founder of DownloadYouthMinistry.com,
youth pastor for thirty years at Saddleback
& Mariners Church, speaker, and author
of 50+ books including *7 Ways to Be Her Hero*

"So many books on this topic are written by people who don't actually interact with real teenagers. But McKee is a practitioner first, a frontline youth worker with *current* and regular interactions with Christian teenagers wrestling with the intersection of their faith and their sexuality. Never condescending to teenagers or parents, Jon brings his blunt and honest writing style to a subject I wish more parents were talking about with their teens."

—Mark Oestreicher, partner, The Youth Cartel and author,
A Parent's Guide to Understanding Teenage Brains
and several other books for parents

"Jonathan McKee's book helps us to remember that 'the talk' is a myth at best, and a terrible strategy at worst. A lifestyle of preparation, a strategic series of discussions, and a proactive commitment to conversation is what our kids need, and this book will help any parent to walk with their kids in confidence."

—Chap Clark, professor of youth, family and culture,
Fuller Theological Seminary

"Jonathan McKee empowers parents with extreme hope and practical help to connect with their teens about this important subject. The valuable tools found in *More Than Just The Talk* are both profound and engaging, helping us keep current in our conversations with our kids! This is a powerful resource for parents, mentors, and pastors who value authentic family life and refuse to settle for surface relationships."

—Bob and Audrey Meisner, bestselling authors,
Marriage Under Cover and TV hosts, *My New Day*

"Our kids have questions about sex—lots of them. But who can they go to for truth? Answer: YOU! Parents have the greatest influence on their children's lives, and next to leading them to faith in Christ, it's your job to help them set godly standards for sex and relationships. This book delivers. It takes the stress out of otherwise awkward conversations and shows you how to make 'the talk' an ongoing, *healthy* dialogue."

—Michael Ross, bestselling author and a former youth editor
at Focus on the Family

"Parents must help their teenagers navigate a sexually charged, often misinformed world by establishing regular open dialogue. In *More Than Just The Talk* Jonathan McKee provides excellent discussion starters and a framework for rooting these conversations of faith and sexuality between parents and their teenagers in their shared faith in Jesus."

—Adam McLane, partner, The Youth Cartel and coauthor,
A Parent's Guide to Understanding Social Media

"Jonathan Mckee is spot on in his new book encouraging parents to become their kids' go-to for information surrounding the topics of sex."

—Craig Gross, founder of XXXchurch.com and iParent.tv,
author of *Touchy Subjects*

MORE THAN JUST THE TALK

Books by Jonathan McKee

FROM BETHANY HOUSE PUBLISHERS

Get Your Teenager Talking

More Than Just "The Talk"

Sex Matters

MORE THAN JUST THE TALK

BECOMING YOUR KIDS' GO-TO PERSON ABOUT

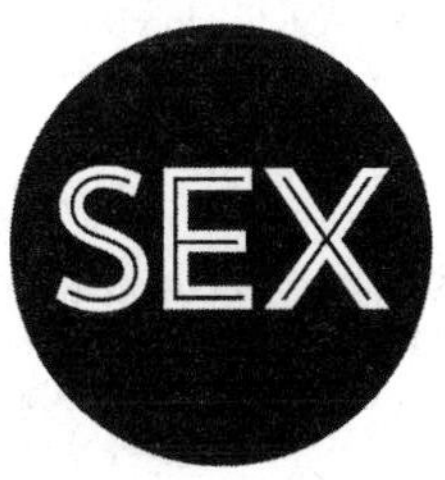

JONATHAN McKEE

BETHANY HOUSE PUBLISHERS
a division of Baker Publishing Group
Minneapolis, Minnesota

Published by Bethany House Publishers
11400 Hampshire Avenue South
Bloomington, Minnesota 55438
www.bethanyhouse.com

Bethany House Publishers is a division of
Baker Publishing Group, Grand Rapids, Michigan

Printed in the United States of America

Library of Congress Cataloging-in-Publication Data is on file at the Library of Congress, Washington, DC.

ISBN 978-0-7642-1294-9

Some names and details have been changed to protect the privacy of those whose stories appear in this book.

Cover design by Greg Jackson, Thinkpen Design, Inc.

Author is represented by WordServe Literary Group.

15 16 17 18 19 20 21 7 6 5 4 3 2 1

In keeping with biblical principles of creation stewardship, Baker Publishing Group advocates the responsible use of our natural resources. As a member of the Green Press Initiative, our company uses recycled paper when possible. The text paper of this book is composed in part of post-consumer waste.

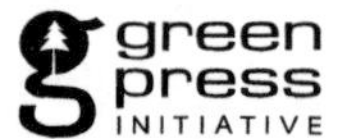

Contents

Acknowledgments

I don't think I've ever requested as much feedback from friends as I did with this book and its counterpart, *Sex Matters*, the corresponding book for teens. This subject always catalyzes a wide array of responses, so I solicited the help of numerous friends, other authors, parents, and youth workers to help me ensure a message relevant to today's parents and then to today's young people.

Thanks to Brian Berry, Pete Sutton, and my brother Thom, who all poured over these books in detail, offering helpful feedback and tweaks. Thanks to Julie Smith, Sande Quattlebaum, Jennifer Smith, Rick Nier, and Joe and Kerry Vivian. Your insights as parents were extremely helpful. Thanks to so many of my blog readers at Jonathan McKeeWrites.com who sent in common questions they hear from young people. And thanks to the many friends and colleagues in the field of parenting and youth ministry who read this book and offered the kind endorsements you see in the first few pages.

Thanks to my friend and agent Greg Johnson from WordServe for making this project happen. Thanks to Andy, Carra, Ellen, and the entire team at Bethany for your hard work on these books, helping make them practical tools to put in the hands of young people, parents, and youth workers.

And thanks mostly to my family for supporting me through this project, putting up with my endless questions and prodding about the subject. You guys rock!

But anything truly good that appears on these pages is from God, who deserves all the credit. God, thanks for your amazing design of sex and intimacy! It's mind-boggling why we constantly mess it up. Thanks for enduring with us when we do. We don't deserve your undeniable love and grace.

Start Here

Unanswered Questions

"How do we know hooking up is really wrong, and even if it is . . . can't I just get forgiveness afterward?"

That was her first question of many, verbatim. She wasn't very articulate, but there was no misunderstanding what this young lady was really asking.

She was sixteen years old going on twenty, wearing tiny little booty shorts and a low-cut blouse exposing the top of her bra and way too much cleavage. She had hugged every guy who entered the room that evening—including adult leaders, with an embrace just a little too long to be comfortable.

Just another night at church youth group.

After twenty years of youth ministry I wish I could tell you this was an isolated incident. Sadly, this scene was all too familiar.

I met her and her friends last September when I spoke to this particular group. A handful of teenagers approached me afterward with questions. She was the second one to talk with me.

I had seen her playing pool with her friends before I spoke. She was the exact same age as my youngest daughter, a frightening thought. In the thirty minutes I observed, I heard her mention a sexually charged TV show and a popular sexually explicit music video that was currently number one on the charts, and watched her make gestures with a pool cue that would have made her mother pass out.

Funny thing . . . she really didn't stick out in this crowd of church kids. The two other girls standing around the pool table were dressed the same way and engaging in similar conversation—that is . . . when they actually talked. Today's conversation between teenagers seems to be only a few sentences at a time, broken with long pauses to check their phones, type something quickly, then resume paying attention to the less important audience . . . *the people in the same room with them.*

A few young men lurked nearby, one with headphones around his neck, another leaning close and sharing an earbud with a girl standing next to him. I didn't hear every song or artist they played, but in the short time I was there, I heard three sexually explicit songs I recognized from the top of the music charts.

I asked the youth pastor a little about these particular teenagers. The sixteen-year-old girl was an elder's daughter, and the young man listening to explicit music was the pastor's son.

Cliché? Maybe. But sadly, a true story.

I wish I could tell you this was a snapshot of today's young people in general, but it's not. It's an accurate picture of today's church kids. If you want to see today's young people, go to a school rally or chaperone a homecoming dance. Scarier yet, find an opportunity to be a fly on the wall when a teenager is traversing virtual hangouts like Tinder or Omegle (both social media sites parents don't want to discover their kids navigating). You'll quickly discover that the antics I saw around the pool table that night were more *Sesame Street* compared to a lot of what's out there.

Sadly, a great chasm is growing between parents and their kids. Most parents have no idea what their kids are downloading and watching, or the kind of conversations they are engaging in each day. Young people stealthily float under the radar, taking full advantage of this disconnect. As a result, the people who abound in misinformation are the ones filling our kids' ears constantly, and the people who know the truth often only engage in mere minutes of healthy conversation each week.

No wonder the Centers for Disease Control has reported that 64.1 percent of seniors in high school have already had sex.[1]

If only someone had told them the explicit truth.

Yes, I realize most parents have attempted "the sex talk" at least once, usually when the school is about to teach sex ed or the neighbor girl gets pregnant.

Pause for a moment and reflect honestly. When did you last talk openly and candidly about sex with your kids? Do you think you answered all their questions? What about the embarrassing questions they were too afraid to ask?

Is oral sex okay since it's not really "sex"?

Why would God make something as good as sex and then just ban it from us?

Is it okay to masturbate if I think about my future spouse when I'm doing it?

How far can I actually go with my boyfriend/girlfriend?

Is living together okay? Isn't marriage a little outdated?

What about same-sex relationships? Since when does God deny any kind of true love?

Have your own kids asked you any of these questions?

Yeah . . . I didn't have the guts to ask my parents many of these questions either.

But in my last two decades of hanging out with teenagers, I've been asked every one of these questions countless times by young people.

A Trail of Hurt

Let me be the first to tell you that my past isn't close to perfect in the area of sex and dating. I left a trail of hurt behind me in high school and college. I still look back in regret for some of the things I did—the consequences are still there.

I wish I had known the truth.

I'm not making excuses; I sincerely wish someone would have told me the whole truth about sex when I was a teenager. Oh, sure, my parents told me all about the birds and the bees when I was growing up. And my dad would have probably answered my questions . . . *had I asked him.*

Did you ask your mom or dad?

Exactly.

So questions remained.

Sure, I took sex education in school. We learned all about the sperm swimming down the birth canal and fighting other sperm to get to that egg. The teacher (I believe he was also the driving instructor) taught us the official names of all the body parts. I was always just wishing he would show more pictures.

We learned about all those diseases—STDs. We saw pictures of open sores like chancres and venereal warts (not quite what I had in mind for pictures). Then I remember hearing about a few infections that could live on a toilet seat for up to two hours (remember those scare tactics?). You can bet that I was making some jumbo toilet-paper nests in public bathrooms after that. But my questions were far from answered.

At church, I remember my youth pastor talking about sex. He said sex was wrong before marriage and he always used that word I hated . . . *petting*. I don't like using a word to describe something sexual that also describes what I do to my dog. And frankly, when adults used irrelevant words from a different era, it only seemed to perpetuate what I already believed: *These adults don't understand my world.*

So . . . questions remained.

No one ever explained to me exactly what the Bible said about sex. I was pretty sure that it was wrong before marriage, but I couldn't really name the verse—and besides, it was just talking about intercourse, right? So I could do everything else? Second and third base were fair game . . . right?

I wanted answers.

Or did I?

I read about sex in every article, book, or magazine I could get my hands on looking for answers. Was I just curious? I can honestly say I wanted to know the truth, but at the same time, I was pretty happy rounding the bases as long as I avoided home plate.

I knew in my heart this was wrong, but no one dared to reveal the explicit details about God's design for sex, even though the Bible was full of explicit details.

As I look back on my life, I have no greater regrets than how I behaved sexually before I was married. If I could change one thing about my past, I would remain sexually pure before marriage.

The blame rests on me, but I really wish someone would have clearly communicated three facts I never understood:

1. Sex is good, and God gave it to us to enjoy. It's not bad or evil; it's not something to be ashamed of; it's an amazing gift given for you to enjoy with someone you don't intend to ever leave . . . *your spouse*. It's better than any hookup you can imagine.
2. This amazing gift of sexual intimacy is more than just "going all the way." It's a passionate journey that begins with intimate touch, peaks when two people have sexual intercourse, and includes everything in between.
3. Pornography and sexually charged entertainment media provoke lust, and lusting is just like committing adultery against our spouse someday. We need to flee any temptations that cause us to lust or engage in sexual immorality.

I wish I had known these things to be true, but I didn't. Sure, I had heard pieces of these truths, but no one ever told me in a language I could understand. Nobody answered all my questions.

If only someone had been bold enough to tell me *the explicit truth*.

The Explicit Truth

Fast-forward to today, and the situation is far scarier. Today, the world abounds in explicit lies. Teenagers have easy access to copious amounts of misinformation emanating from every screen and each circle of friends they encounter. This is frightening for me as a parent of three.

Where can they hear the truth?

Who is going to answer their questions? MTV? YouTube? Ask.fm?

The fact is, I had questions when I was in high school, in a world where 1 in 18 teenagers in America had a sexually transmitted disease.[2]

Now 1 in 4 American teenage girls has an STD,[3] the two biggest being HPV and chlamydia. HPV is not only the number one sexually transmitted infection in the United States, it is the number one cause for cervical cancer in women.[4] Chlamydia is virtually asymptomatic, so it often stays under the radar and spreads from person to person without their knowledge. If undetected, this STD often leads to pelvic inflammatory disease, a known cause for infertility in women.[5]

Do you think this is information our kids should know about? Who is going to tell our kids *the truth*?

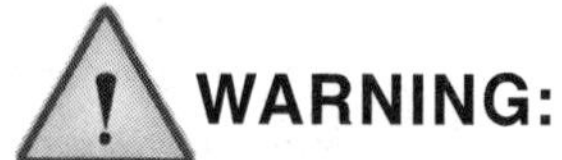

WARNING:

The purpose of this book is to help parents explain the *explicit truth* in a world full of explicit lies. Sadly, when you and your children walk into the grocery store or big-box store this week, you'll probably hear some of those lies leaking through the speakers and see them poking out of the magazine racks to your right and left at the checkout counter. In fact, unless you literally lock your kids in the basement, never to leave the house (which I don't recommend, by the way), they will be exposed to sexually charged media messages . . . and these messages aren't typically recommending "*Wait until marriage for sex.*"

In this book, especially in the initial chapters, I'm going to be giving you a peek at some of the common messages our kids hear. And let me warn you, when you read some of the lyrics and hear some of the lies so commonplace in today's world, some of you are going to be offended. And if you are offended . . . *good!* You should be offended. Because these are the lies our world offers in abundance.

So keep reading, because this book doesn't focus on the lies. In fact, the majority of the book focuses on the truth.

Let's start by taking note of some of the loud voices our kids are hearing day to day.

1

The Loud Voices

"Of course you should do it."

"I'm just gonna move my family to Amish Pennsylvania!"

I had heard it countless times from parents tired of the infiltration of raunchy messages from entertainment media. Was Pennsylvania's Lancaster County truly a Utopia paved with purity and innocence?

One day I received a call from a church in Lancaster County. "Can you please come speak to our church about parenting this smartphone generation?" For about thirty minutes I talked with the leaders from this very conservative Mennonite Brethren church. I thoroughly enjoyed the conversation. They were biblically solid and culturally aware, but apparently they were experiencing struggles very similar to what parents were experiencing all across the U.S.

A few months later I flew across the country from my home in California to Amish Pennsylvania to finally see this perceived mecca of virtue and incorruptibility with my own two eyes. I'll never forget the drive from my hotel to the church in my small rental car. Within minutes I was following a buggy along the smooth paved road.

Soon, I was in line behind three horse-drawn buggies. (I snapped a quick pic and sent it to my kids back home.)

Eventually I arrived at the church. I wore a jacket and tie that particular morning, despite the American church's growing trend toward jeans and a polo. As much as I liked to dress casual, this was the East Coast, and this church was ultra conservative. My hunch was correct. The first three teenagers I encountered were dressed in either slacks and a tie or a dress. The men were in suits. A few women actually wore head covers.

As I watched my audience arrive, I began to wonder about the sermon I had planned for the morning service. I was going to preach about Acts 17, sharing how the apostle Paul used the culture around him to springboard conversations about the Gospel with the people of Athens.

I quickly checked in with the church leaders who had brought me out. "Are you sure you want me to talk about today's culture?" I leaned in really close, thinking out loud. "That lady in the third row has a doily on her head."

They chuckled. "Yeah, our church is pretty conservative, but they are experiencing most of the struggles you have been talking about in your parenting articles and your blog recently. So please, give it to them. Tell them the unedited truth."

I shrugged my shoulders. "All right."

I was impressed. Often, churches have a false sense of security and think, *Not our kids*. This church seemed to realize how susceptible they were to the world's influence.

As I began speaking to the conservative congregation, I showed them the top ten songs young people were listening to across the country. The number one song on the charts that day opened with the lyrics, "Wakin' up in the mornin', two hoes layin' next to me."[1]

I glanced at the lady in the third row with the head cover. Her eyes had grown as big as saucers.

I spent the next thirty minutes giving the church an accurate peek through the porthole of youth culture, and then proposed we follow the apostle Paul's example of interacting about the culture instead of overreacting to it. The church was responsive as a whole, but my eyes kept wandering over to the lady in the third row. She looked . . . *angry*.

After I finished speaking, sure enough, she walked right up to me with a scowl on her face. I thought, *Oh boy. Here goes!*

The first words out of her mouth shocked me. She simply said, "Thank you."

My thoughts were, *You're welcome . . . but please tell that to your face*.

Before I had a chance to respond, she went on. "My kids hear that music all the time."

I was truly surprised. "Really? Here in Lancaster County?"

"Yes. Whodathunkit," she said, smiling for a brief second. She glanced over her shoulder and lowered her volume just a notch. "My fifth-grader goes to the local public school. During art class, his teacher lets the kids play all the 'clean' versions." She made little quote marks with her fingers when she said the word *clean*.

"What songs do they play?" I asked, truly curious.

"All of those," she said, pointing to the screen where I had just posted the lyrics of many of the current top ten songs.

Lancaster County.

Whodathunkit?

Let's face it. The world isn't G-rated. When we roll our carts to the checkout counter at the corner grocery store, we are forced to navigate a gauntlet of magazine images seeped in sexuality. Do you think our kids don't see headlines like "Try a Threesome to Spice up Your Marriage" or "Ten Ways to Please Your Boyfriend in Bed"?

Wander over to the book section next time you're in Costco. Why shouldn't our daughters pick up the newest attempt at *Fifty Shades of Grey*? Their twenty-seven-year-old Freshman English teacher is reading it. Raunchy entertainment media is part of the staple diet of the Millennial generation, those in their twenties and early thirties. Consider Millennial role models Chelsea Handler and Tucker Max, for example. Both of them helped make blunt and raunchy popular nearly a decade ago, and both appeared in *Vulture*'s recent list of "100 Pop-Culture Things That Make You a Millennial." Salon describes them like this:

> These two raunch-masters arrived on the scene at just about the same time—Chelsea Handler in 2005 with her first book *My Horizontal Life: A Collection of One-Night Stands* and Tucker Max in 2006 with *I Hope They Serve Beer in Hell*. Both made their mark by dishing about their sex lives, and generally being offensive and "real." *The New York Times* validated Max by essentially dubbing him the inventor of a genre called "fratire." Television validated Handler by giving her a show on E! And both showed us that being disgusting was as valid a path to success as anything else these days.[2]

Does this kind of raunch and crude sexual talk seep into our homes? Do you ever turn on the TV? When my dad grew up, families watched *Leave It to Beaver*. When I was a teenager, families watched *The Cosby Show*. What is the norm for families now . . . *Family Guy*? As a dad of three kids—seventeen, nineteen, and twenty-one as I write this, I can't help but worry about what they are gleaning from media entertainment today.

And I haven't even addressed all the distractions available through the phones in our kids' pockets. My guess is most kids aren't spending the majority of their time on their Bible apps.

Hope for the Best

How are most parents responding to this influx of lies in our kids' world?

The majority just hope for the best.

I wish I were making this up. McAfee recently published a study about young people's online behavior. In this report, 69 percent of the young people surveyed admitted they take measures to hide their online behavior from their parents.[3]

I'm sure these parents would do something about this if they only knew . . . *right?*

Sadly, the same study revealed that "74% of parents say they don't have the time or the energy to keep up with everything their child is doing online," and "72% of parents say they are overwhelmed by modern technology and just hope for the best."[4]

Hope for the best?

Is that really all parents can do?

Maybe we need to start paying attention to what our kids are absorbing. Scratch out the word *maybe* there. Point of fact: Your pediatrician would tell you to start devoting full attention to these entertainment media messages. So would the doctors who engage in Kaiser Family Foundation's huge entertainment media study every five years. In fact, in one of their studies of the effects of entertainment media in the lives of eight- to eighteen-year-olds, they concluded:

> This generation truly is the media generation, devoting more than a quarter of each day to media. As media devices become increasingly portable, and as they spread even further through young people's environments . . . media messages will become an even more ubiquitous presence in an already media-saturated world. Anything that takes up this much space in young people's lives deserves our full attention.[5]

Doctors' orders. Are you "giving your full attention"?

Let's take just a glimpse at some of these loud voices in our kids' ears, specifically music, video games, television, and the Internet.

Music

Every generation has had song lyrics that pushed the envelope. But of late, that envelope is no longer pushed; it's wide open with someone begging you to look in.

Sexual messages are a common theme in today's music—and not just a few obscure songs, but often the most popular songs on the charts. Let me give you a few glaring examples from the last decade. One is Robin Thicke's "Blurred Lines," a song many remember because of his scandalous performance with Miley Cyrus at the MTV Video Music Awards in 2013. The song spent twelve weeks at the top of the Billboard Hot 100 chart. Thicke's message about women in this song is clear as he repeatedly says, "I know you want it."

When rapper T.I. joins Thicke at the mic in this song, the already offensive lyrics decline. He calls women degrading names and describes sex in very raunchy terms. Google "Robin Thicke Blurred Lines lyrics" to peek at what the song is communicating.

The music video matched the vile lyrics, with topless girls dancing around provocatively in nothing more than G-strings. This racy video was so successful, it's burned into the memories of teens. It rode the number one spot on the iTunes charts for more than three months. Most parents didn't realize any kid with iTunes on their smartphone had topless women and disgusting lyrics just a click away in the top ten for almost a year. The same video also drew over 100 million views on Vevo's music video page in just a few months' time.

But it doesn't take nudity to make a video sexually explicit. In fact, you don't even need the "explicit" label to make a song explicit. Take Flo Rida's song "Whistle," for example. I don't know what's more pathetic, the fact that a song about oral sex went number one on the charts back in 2012, or the fact that people argued this song was clean.

The song was number one for several months that year, topped the iTunes charts, and became the number one ringtone that people downloaded on their cell phones.

Artists today have mastered the craft of making sexually provocative songs and music videos under the guise of "clean." "Whistle" doesn't have any swear words, so it's not tagged with an explicit label. Parents who aren't savvy to what pop culture is offering don't realize that their kids are walking around listening to racy music for literally several hours a day.

Of course, when we talk to most young people about sexually charged music and images like this, the majority of them respond, "This stuff doesn't affect me."

Experts would not agree.

The journal *Pediatrics* released a study a few years ago revealing the obvious: "Teens whose iPods are full of music with raunchy, sexual lyrics start having sex sooner than those who prefer other songs." The study was very specific:

> Teens who said they listened to lots of music with degrading sexual messages were almost twice as likely to start having intercourse or

> other sexual activities within the following two years as were teens who listened to little or no sexually degrading music. Among heavy listeners, 51 percent started having sex within two years, versus 29 percent of those who said they listened to little or no sexually degrading music.[6]

But the infiltration of sexually charged entertainment media isn't limited to what is coming through our kids' headphones.

Video Games

In a country where over 90 percent of young people between the ages of two and seventeen are playing video games,[7] it's hard to ignore what they encounter on those platforms—especially considering every time a new *Grand Theft Auto* game is released, it immediately jumps to the number one spot. Kids can't get enough of this M-rated game.

What's so scary about one video game?

In September 2013, when *Grand Theft Auto* 5 was released, it broke all the sales records, raking in 1 billion dollars in the first three days. Young gamers couldn't stop talking about it. Like its predecessors, this game made every effort to maximize the M rating. Your character can go into a strip club and watch strippers remove their tops while giving you a lap dance. You can also pick up a hooker, choose three types of sex with her—oral, anal, or vaginal—and then choose a weapon to kill her with when you're done so you can get your money back. In most screen recordings you find online, the player just ran over her with his car multiple times, literally backing over her when he was through with her. Most players we viewed online were laughing while doing this.

What kind of sex are these young people learning?

Do you think Mom really knows what they're playing?

Some parents think, *My kid would never play a game like that*. That's exactly what my friend John thought. And he was right. His sixteen-year-old daughter, Elise, wouldn't play a game like that. But when she and her friend went to their friend Josh's house, Josh and his friend Chris were sitting in the living room wearing headsets and playing it.

Elise knew Josh from her church.

Elise didn't pay much attention at first, but when she saw a guy having sex with a girl right there on the screen, she took off Josh's headset and asked him, "What the heck are you guys playing?"

Josh claimed, "Oh, I just ignore these parts. I need the points real quick." This wasn't his first time playing the series. In past *Grand Theft Auto* games, characters could restore their health to 100 percent when they had sex with a prostitute.

Josh's mom didn't have a clue what he was playing.

The games in the *Grand Theft Auto* series aren't the only sexually explicit games (they just happen to be the fastest-selling game on the shelf every time they are released). Popular games like *Far Cry, God of War, Red Dead Redemption*, and the *Hitman* series all have sexual content as well.

Whenever I ask young gamers what they think of the sex and violence in games, they always defend the game, responding, "I don't really pay attention to all that sex and violence, I just love the gameplay!"

Funny, that's similar to what they say about the TV shows they are watching.

Television

Young people are soaking in TV at a rate of two to four and a half hours a day, depending on who you ask. The Kaiser Family Foundation's entertainment media study, frequently cited by the most respected medical journals, revealed that eight- to eighteen-year-olds devote four hours and twenty-nine minutes per day to television programming.[8]

Some parents might claim, "But my kid never sits down in front of the TV." They don't have to. Most of us have given them a handheld device where they can stream their favorite programming via Hulu, Netflix, or numerous other sources.

So what are they seeing?

Sex and nudity is becoming much more prominent on TV. Most television gets away with this by using blurred, pixelated, and cleverly covered nudity. Many will be quick to tell you pixelated nudity "isn't really nudity" . . . *as if nudity were the only concern.*

But this blurred nudity debate is only about broadcast television, which is a rather humorous debate when 91 percent of American homes pay for TV.[9] When I grew up, TV meant NBC, CBS, ABC, and maybe Fox if you had a really good antenna. Now it's not uncommon for homes to subscribe to HBO, Cinemax, or Showtime. After all, many cable and satellite companies throw in these channels free or at a discount for a limited time to entice customers to keep these channels, where sex and nudity are commonplace. All three of these channels provide soft-core porn on most given evenings.

Some of the most popular shows exist on these pay channels. *Entertainment Weekly* recently posted their esteemed 100 all-time greatest TV shows ever, where HBO earned two slots in the top ten, including the number one spot. Series like *Game of Thrones*, *Sex and the City*, *The Sopranos*, and other HBO shows all made the top 100.[10]

Game of Thrones, one of the most popular shows for young Millennials, is so graphic with sex and nudity that *Saturday Night Live* even did a spoof about the show, claiming it was written by a thirteen-year-old boy who made sure "there were lots of boobs in the show." *SNL* questioned the reasoning behind a scene in an episode where a guy is receiving oral sex while peeking through a peephole watching another couple have sex. It's not uncommon for *Game of Thrones'* fans to see full frontal nudity of both men and women during an episode, and see several minutes of sex scenes, including lesbian sex scenes and/or threesomes. The only difference between this show and hard-core porn is the lack of extreme close-ups.

Yet if you turn on *Good Morning America*, don't be surprised when you find Robin Roberts openly talk about watching last night's episode of *Game of Thrones*. America can't get enough of this show.

U.S. audiences seem to be less and less concerned about sexually explicit material. After all, it's in their favorite shows.

In my research for this book, I interviewed literally hundreds of young people. Whenever the subject of these pay channels came up, I'd ask, "So, did you ever find the late-night programming on these channels distracting?"

I received a variety of answers. Here's the gist of some of the more common answers I received from different *Christian* young people:

> "Yeah, I never watched them regularly, but sometimes I'd be channel-flipping and I'd land on two naked girls on top of each other. It's pretty hard to change the channel at that point."

> "I watched late night Cinemax for about a week and finally realized I needed to tell someone to just block the channel. It was too much of a distraction to even know that channel was available in my house!"

> "Lots of my friends at school would talk about something they saw on HBO or Showtime, like, 'Did you see those two girls going at it on *Californication*?' or 'Did you see what happened on *Masters of Sex*?' It made me curious so I found downloads of episodes online."

Of all the males I asked, not one who had those channels in his house for any amount of time had *not* seen the soft-core porn or after-hours programming the channels offered. I truly searched for the one exception and never found him.

My wife, Lori, and I have noticed the trend toward this sexually charged programming on basic cable channels as well. From A&E to FX, we've encountered sex scenes that made us look at each other and ask, "What on earth are we watching here?" Last month we were watching a cop drama on FX. A man got into a car with a woman to negotiate some illegal activity they were planning, and the woman took off her top, spread her legs (wearing just a bra and a skirt at this point), and basically told him they had a deal if he was willing to give her oral sex. His head went down, and then we saw a shot from outside the car of her legs sticking out of the window. The channel got away with this scene because it never actually showed full breasts or genitals, but showed more than enough for your imagination to take over. The go-to sex scene for these channels is often two completely naked people on top of each other, with only backs, bare bottoms, and sides visible.

This is basic cable.

If full frontal nudity is the only prohibition, then you're going to encounter sexually explicit entertainment every day you turn on the TV or open a magazine.

Needless to say, Lori and I decided that this show probably wasn't one we should be watching, not just because of its nudity quota, but because we were concerned about media glamorizing cheap, random sexual encounters. It was frustrating because we were really starting to enjoy the show, but it was featuring these kinds of gratuitous sex scenes more and more.

So is TV as a whole growing more risqué?

Back in April 2013, the FCC posted a public notice about considering allowing more nudity and expletives on television.[11] The public expressed overwhelming outrage, with 95,000 comments. But compare that to the literally millions of viewers who watch episodes of *Game of Thrones* each week.

Does America really object?

Of course, young people will claim that watching sexually charged TV or movies doesn't affect them negatively. And again, experts wouldn't agree.

A recent study in the journal *Psychological Science* revealed that promiscuous programming promotes real-life promiscuity. Young teenagers who are exposed to more sexual content in movies start having sex at younger ages, have more sexual partners, and engage in riskier sexual activities. In fact:

> Young teens who viewed movies with sexual content were profoundly influenced by what they watched. They initiated sexual behavior earlier than their peers who had viewed less sexual content, and they tended to imitate the on-screen sexual behaviors they saw—which included casual sex, having multiple partners and high-risk behaviors.[12]

A *Washington Times* article reporting the above study observed, "It's not surprising, really. Teens crave information about sex—and too often turn to the media for information."[13]

But the TV screen isn't the only place where young people are absorbing misinformation about sex.

The Internet

Facebook, Instagram, YouTube . . . what are young people gleaning from these sources where they often spend several hours per day? And let's be honest—does their web browsing stop at social networking?

Parents shudder at the thought of their kids viewing pornography, but sadly, Internet porn is becoming more and more difficult for kids to miss (that's why I've devoted an entire chapter to helping our kids resist the lure of pornography—chapter 9).

- The average age of first Internet exposure to pornography is eleven.[14]
- Twenty-eight percent of sixteen- to seventeen-year-olds have been unintentionally exposed to porn online.[15]
- Eighty-three percent of boys and 57 percent of girls have seen group sex online.[16]

Jamila Rizvi, editor of the online women's site Mamamia, noticed the power of porn in the life of teenagers:

> One of the things with the accessibility of the Internet is that porn is easy to get . . . it's a click of a button away. So you've got 10-, 11-, 12-year-old girls, and importantly boys seeing women behaving in a particular way and they think that's normal. There's an element of imitation, that's what you do when you're a 'tween or a teen. You're learning to become an adult so you look at the adults around you and you look at the adults on the computer.[17]

Even teenagers who aren't frequenting porn are navigating an online world with those who are. The effects of porn are seeping into the communication young people are engaging in on social media sites. Sixteen-year-old Olympia Nelson speaks about this sexualized world of social media in her frank article, "Dark Undercurrents of Teenage Girls' Selfies":

> Seeing some of these images can feel too intimate. It's almost as though we're peering through a window. Some photos may be of girls showing skin, or girls lying on a bed. Just about all are seeking some sort of approval from their friends. The aim is not to communicate joy but to score a position. . . . The aesthetic yardstick is what they see in pornography. So girls have to conform to what boys see in pornography. And then girls post photos to "out-hot" the other girls by porn star criteria.[18]

If you've ever navigated through the teen world of social media, you've seen it. Even the most innocent of girls are caving to the pressure to be sexy and take selfies wearing a shirt with a plunging neckline, not just because Taylor Swift wore one, but because it's a sure way to be noticed and to get "likes."

Who doesn't want to be "liked"?

Smartphones

And what about the little device in our kids' pockets? They are used by most Americans over two and a half hours a day.[19]

What messages are your kids gleaning from their phones?

When I walk on a high school campus, I don't have to look far to see teenagers with their heads down, engrossed in the two-inch screen they hold in their hands. This little device can be used for all kinds of good. It can help them become better organized, keep up with positive friends, and even communicate with family. But sadly, this little tool can also open the door to plenty of distractions in a young person's life, often ending in disaster.

So what happens when catastrophe strikes? Teenagers believe the lies from all these loud voices, and many of them make costly mistakes.

How should parents respond?

How do parents typically respond when these poor decisions come to light?

The easiest and most common reaction is *overreaction*. Put your foot through the flat-screen, unplug the Internet, and move to Amish

Pennsylvania. (Oh, that's right . . . Lancaster County parents are going through the same struggles. Maybe move to Kenya?)

If you ever let your kids out of the house (which I recommend, by the way), then they are going to encounter the world's values. We can't protect our kids from every racy image and wayward philosophy they encounter. Those parents who try to swoop down and save their kids from every struggle only cripple their kids from learning to stand on their own.

From Overreaction to Interaction

That's why we need to turn our *overreaction* into *interaction.*

Which do you think works better: flipping out or pausing for a moment, taking a deep breath, and starting a dialogue with our kids about some of these influences when they encounter them?

Parents always tell me, "My kids don't want to talk with me about this stuff."

Perhaps that's because we freak out every time they give us a peek into their world.

What if we stopped *overreacting* and began *interacting* about real-life struggles?

That's the scary part for many parents. We don't even realize what real life is for teenagers today. Some of us would be shocked if we found out.

That's what happened to "Aaron's" mom. She was browsing the family computer, in search of a website she had visited the day before, and found where her sixteen-year-old son, Aaron, had been browsing the night prior. As she saw the images unfold on the screen before her eyes, she burst into tears. She had never seen such perversion before. She could only ask one question: "*Why?*"

Aaron told me that when he arrived home that night, his parents were both waiting up for him. "When I saw them both sitting there together on the couch with the TV off, I knew it was serious.

"My mom was bawling. She just kept asking me, 'Why?'

"I couldn't tell her why," Aaron explained. "The only answer I could muster was, 'I don't know, but I just can't stop.'"

Aaron's mom kept pressing him, trying to find out how he could look at "this filth." Finally Aaron's dad stepped in and did something very wise. He said, "Honey, our son doesn't know why, but he's asking us for help."

What's it going to take for our kids to ask us for help?

If we're willing to sit down and truly listen to our kids, we might discover some unpleasant truths. Are we willing to have those explicit discussions?

I've met countless parents who opened the doors to conversations with their daughter and discovered she was tired of the lies and was desperately looking for truth. Many teenage girls today have bought the lie that being sexy . . . or even giving sex . . . makes them happy. I've met very few who have traveled that path and found happiness.

Donna Freitas, a former professor of religion at Hofstra and Boston Universities, addresses this in her book, *The End of Sex*, which studies the hookup culture on college campuses. She reveals, "Both young women and young men are seriously unhappy with the way things are. It's rare that I find a young woman or a man who says hooking up is the best thing ever."[20]

She goes on to describe sex in the life of the average college kid:

> Sex is something you're not to care about. The reason for hooking up is less about pleasure and fun than performance and gossip—it's being able to update about it. Social media is fostering a very unthinking and unfeeling culture. We're raising our kids to be performers.[21]

The world is screaming lies at our kids.

Are we creating an atmosphere where our kids can open up to us and dialogue about the truth?

Don't Give Up

As a fellow parent with teenagers of my own, let me encourage you, *don't give up*.

As an author who studies parenting and youth culture daily, let me reassure you, *don't give up*.

As a guy who has been hanging with teenagers since way back when they all carried pagers . . . let me inspire you, *don't give up*.

Yes, the messages bombarding our kids every day seem overwhelming. But all the experts agree: Your conversations with your kids about sex make a huge difference. In fact, parents make the biggest impact. So don't be overwhelmed; this book is going to provide you with the encouragement and the tools to engage in these meaningful conversations.

Kids whose parents are hush-hush about these struggles have to figure out the answers somewhere else. Usually, that "somewhere else" is on a glowing screen or in the high school locker room.

Would you rather they hear the truth about sex from you . . . or from *2 Broke Girls*? This popular CBS comedy provides plenty of sexual humor, but doesn't typically address the consequences of living a promiscuous lifestyle.

Are you having these conversations, or are you one of the *quiet voices*? Let's pause and take a quick look at these quiet voices in the next chapter.

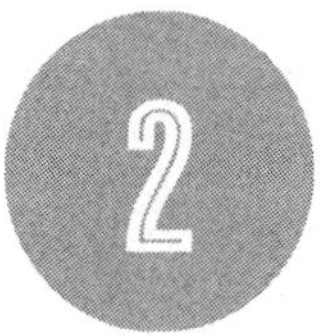

The Quiet Voices

"Shhhh! Don't talk about it!"

Plenty of loud voices are shouting *explicit lies* at our kids.

Where are the voices telling the *explicit truth*?

A few months ago I met a young teen mom who became pregnant during her first year in college, was kicked out of her house, and was forced to have the baby on her own.

She was one of the pastor's daughters.

Everyone in the church knew. Huge ordeal!

Pregnant and with no place to stay, she went to live at a friend of a friend's house. This guy was an alcoholic and let her sleep on the sofa. Needless to say, it was a scary eight months.

After the baby was born, she eventually restored the relationship with her parents and moved back home. She began attending church again, this time with a little baby in her arms.

I met her when her daughter was a toddler. She approached me after my parent workshop and shared her story, giving me just a peek at the day-to-day struggles of a single twenty-year-old mom. As she was reflecting back and telling me about her mistakes, I asked her, "What will you do differently as a parent to help your own kids not make the same mistakes?"

Without hesitation she responded, "I will actually talk about sex! And not just once—*all the time*!"

She glanced over her shoulder, took a step closer, and spoke quietly: "My parents *never* talked about it. My dad *wouldn't* talk about it. He sent my mom into my room once to have 'the talk.' It wasn't enough.

"I had questions, struggles, and desires, and it was painfully obvious that they *didn't* want to talk about it. So I didn't ask them. I found out on my own." She held her baby up as she said that last sentence.

I wish I could tell you this girl's story was an isolated incident. But . . . *I hear this perspective all the time.*

Three weeks ago I met a college kid with a two-year-old son. He was twenty-one years old, working full time, going to school full time . . . and a single dad.

After hearing him share his heart, I asked him the same question: "What would you do to equip your son for these kinds of life decisions?"

He didn't even blink. "I'm going to talk about sex with my son a lot!"

Déjà vu?

He continued, "My dad talked with me about it once. Youth group talked about it once a year, but they never answered my questions."

He gave me specifics. "When I went to college, I would go into my girlfriend's dorm room. I just thought, *This is so cool! This is what happens in every movie!* I didn't think through anything. No one had told me specifically, *'If you get alone with a girl who initiates sex, it will be impossible to stop!'*"

He leaned forward in his chair. "I want my kid to know the truth. I'm going to prepare him for that day so he doesn't have to figure it out on his own."

In 2013 Anne Marie Miller penned the article "3 Things You Don't Know About Your Children and Sex." In her article, this pastor's daughter confessed about her own porn addiction that began when she was a teenager. She had experienced abuse from someone she trusted and didn't know if what he was doing was good or bad. Confused and looking for answers, she turned to the Internet for education. This search quickly led to porn. She writes:

> I was too afraid to ask.
>
> What started as an innocent pursuit of knowledge quickly escalated into a coping mechanism.
>
> When I looked at pornography, I felt a feeling of love and safety—at least for a brief moment. But those brief moments of relief disappeared and I was left even more ashamed and confused than when I started. Pornography provided me both an emotional and a sexual release.
>
> For five years I carried this secret. I was twenty-one when I finally opened up to a friend *only* because she opened up to me first about her struggle with sexual sin.[1]

She had questions but was too afraid to ask.

Are you noticing a pattern here?

Stop Thinking They Aren't Thinking About It

Last year I was speaking at a camp in rural Wisconsin and I brought up the subject of sex to my middle school audience of about five hundred kids. I shared the truth about sex: "It isn't naughty; it isn't bad; it's an amazing gift God gave us to enjoy in marriage someday." I even had them turn to some Scripture on the subject.

Two moms approached me after my talk and pointed at me angrily. "Why are you talking about sex with this age group?!" One mom even said, "These kids aren't even thinking about this yet!"

I tried my best not to drop to the ground in hysterics. Do kids not have TV, Internet, or smartphones in Wisconsin? What did they think guys talked about during PE every day . . . the Packers? (Actually, they might. . . . But they also talk about sex.)

I realize it's hard for parents to hear about the content coming from the loud voices I exposed in the previous chapter. It's no fun reading that 83 percent of boys and 57 percent of girls have seen group sex online.[2] Even if our younger kids haven't thought much about sex yet, they most likely have stumbled upon sexual images or overheard other kids talking about it.

The sad fact is, I've seen examples of these overprotective moms who assert their kids' purity, avoid the conversation, and, too many times to count, their kids end up completely rebelling, getting pregnant, becoming addicted to porn . . . the ending to that story is rarely "happily ever after." Interestingly enough, most of the research on porn reveals that it is actually more prevalent in rural areas, where most moms think their kids aren't affected by it. A cruel irony.

Stop thinking they aren't thinking about it. Chances are, they've thought about it a few times—*or a few times per day*—and they have questions.

I had a similar incident in my hometown. I shared the truth about sex at a large conference with about a thousand teens—youth groups from about seventy churches. I opened up Proverbs 5, an amazing passage showing God's design for sex and how enjoyable it can be. The passage uses the word *breasts*.

After sharing the verse, I watched a youth leader gather up his entire youth group and walk out.

Really?

Did they want me to edit the Bible?

I befriended the youth pastor years later in my seminary class and asked him, "So why did you walk out when I read that passage?"

He shrugged his shoulders. "I don't know. My other leaders just looked at me like I should do something, so we left. It just didn't seem right talking about sex so openly."

Let's face it. It's one of those topics that we don't talk about very often. It just feels . . . *naughty*.

This guy isn't alone. Many people have been raised with a warped sense of puritanical values and mistake *silence* for *purity*. "We don't talk about these things in our house."

Really? Too bad. The Bible does . . . *explicitly*. Try reading the book of Genesis with your ten-year-old. You'll blush more times than you can count.

We need to speak the truth to our kids, and we shouldn't wait until they get their driver's license to engage them in this conversation.

Mark Oestreicher, author of *Understanding Your Young Teen*, argues that middle school is the perfect time to talk with teens about sex. He went as far to say, "It's pure irresponsibility as a youth worker to avoid this subject."[3]

Mark knows sixth-, seventh-, and eighth-grade students are all over the road developmentally. Some think about sex often while others barely fathom it. But honest communication is necessary as they hear about it all around them and questions arise. "In general, most middle schoolers need conversations about what sex will be more than they need conversations about what it already is."[4]

Ignoring it won't make it go away.

Is this silence a national problem?

It just might be *international*!

As I was doing some of this research, my dad was on a mission trip to Uganda, teaching and equipping African pastors to preach God's Word. One of the African ministers traveling with him, Andrew, is a pastor who visits different villages talking about sex and the AIDS pandemic, educating young people with the truth. Sadly, in African cultures, they rarely talk about sex. (*Wow, Uganda is just like Wisconsin!*) Andrew has built trust with several of the schools and has been teaching "True Love Waits" rallies, presenting the truth and then interacting with kids afterward, answering the many questions they have.

My dad sent me the following email from his phone while in Uganda:

> Had another good night's sleep. We are at a Catholic retreat center and it is pretty primitive, but the team is all so positive. We don't have showers or hot water. Learning to wash my hair at a faucet. Cold shaves.
>
> Our team that taught the "True Love Waits" to 200 middle school kids was pretty moving yesterday. After Andrew made the AIDS presentation, they handed out cards for questions. Everyone wrote questions. Schools are in English. The questions were heart-wrenching.

Things like, "I've been raped. How do I know if I have AIDS?" Or "I have AIDS. Should I quit having sex with my boyfriend?" This from 12- and 13-year-olds!

The headmaster of the school invited them back today to talk to another 200 kids. The team is very excited to present this material that Andrew has written. He was on a Ministry of Education committee when he wrote this, and now he can present this in public schools.

The African AIDS epidemic is pretty scary. I've spoken to thousands of kids in Uganda for the last couple years and have seen it with my own eyes. One of the church events I spoke at provided free AIDS tests. It was the first time I spoke where my talk was followed up with an announcement to remember to pick up your HIV test results.

Those of us in the U.S. would like to think that we have an entire ocean separating us from this problem, but sadly, this isn't just an African problem. Remember, it was only a few years ago that Americans woke up to the headline, "One in Four Teen Girls Has an STD."[5]

Perhaps American parents need to have more conversations about sex.

The Void of Truth

Silence only breeds ignorance. *U.S. News* recently wrote about a study revealing that 24 percent of teenage girls who took the human papillomavirus (HPV) vaccine mistakenly thought their risk of getting other STDs was lowered.[6] Sound crazy? I constantly encountered this kind of reasoning in my work with middle school students on campuses.

"I'll just wear two condoms."

"I always just shower really good after sex."

The fact is, parents aren't talking about sex frequently enough with their kids. One sex talk isn't enough. This needs to be an ongoing conversation!

The journal *Pediatrics* published a study entitled "Beyond the 'Big Talk,'" encouraging parents to consider having repeated discussions with their children about many aspects of sex instead of just one "big talk." The conclusion of the study was simple: "The more parents talked with their children, the closer their relationships." In fact, the relationship between parent and child really benefitted "when the discussions moved beyond 'safe' or impersonal subjects such as puberty, reproduction and sexually transmitted diseases to more private topics such as masturbation and how sex feels."

Perhaps "explicit" isn't so bad when it's true.

The above report "cited earlier studies that showed children who were communicated with were more likely to delay intercourse and, if they chose to have sex, to use contraception and have fewer partners."[7] I don't know about you, but to me, these conversations sound worth the effort.

I talk about sex to young people frequently, openly, honestly, and explicitly, but I'm never graphic for the sake of being graphic. TV and movies feature sexual content frequently, but they often use sex as a lure for viewers. They get graphic because people want to see graphic. Most of us are familiar with the term "sex sells."

But often, TV doesn't tell the whole story. That's where parents can make a difference. If our kids are exposed to these messages, we can *finish the story*.

Last year I spoke to a group of parents about how to respond to our teenagers if we discover they have been watching or listening to raunchy entertainment media. At the time, Nicki Minaj had a song in the top 100 titled "High School." The music video was readily clickable in the top ten of iTunes and Spotify on most teenagers' phones, and the song was getting airplay everywhere. (I actually heard it on the radio when I was in Kampala, Uganda.) To parents' surprise, I had just heard a teenager playing the song in youth group, so I used it as an example of how to respond to our teenagers.

In this song, Nicki talks about sex explicitly, as she does in many songs. In one part of the song she mentions not having sex (using the f-word) with "beginners" but instead letting them touch her genitals. (Feel free to Google "Nicki Minaj 'High School' lyrics" if you'd like to see exactly how she words it.) Nicki describes explicit sexual acts often in her songs. In 2014 she did it again with her chart-topping hits "Anaconda" and "Bang Bang."

Parents are, of course, horrified when they hear these raunchy lyrics. When they heard that one of these songs was played by one of their own kids, they became distressed.

At this point in my parent workshop, I shared some Scripture with them. As I had with the Mennonites in Lancaster County, I shared the story in Acts 17, where the apostle Paul wanted to reach out to the people of Athens. In this passage we see him walk around the city and look at their idols. When he saw their idols, he "was distressed to see that the city was full of idols" (Acts 17:16 NIV). I encouraged these parents: "It's okay to feel distressed when we take a peek at the culture our kids are living in." "It's okay to feel distressed when you hear Nicki's lyrics." But then I asked the parents an important question: *"When we feel distressed, how should we respond?"*

Turning back to the Scripture, we see Paul initiate discussion with the people about what he saw. In fact, he uses what he noticed about the idols as a springboard to talk about the Gospel. He basically says, "You guys are really religious. You worship a lot of gods. In fact, you even worship an idol you label as 'an unknown god.' Funny . . . I know who that is. Let me tell you about Him!" (see vv. 22–23). Then Paul introduced them to the real God. He even quoted some of their pagan poets' "lyrics" in his description of God.

Imagine if parents were so shrewd. Instead of overreacting when we hear our kids listening to foul lyrics like this, what if we addressed those lyrics with some questions that made our kids think?

> *"So why is it that Nicki is saying she lets guys touch her like this in this song?"*
>
> *"Is it okay for a guy to touch his girlfriend like this? Why or why not?"*
>
> *"What does the Bible say about this?"*

Yes, we might need to set some realistic boundaries so our thirteen-year-olds learn that lyrics like that are unhealthy and don't belong on their phones. But we also shouldn't be afraid to talk candidly about the subject, sharing the truth on the matter. We won't even get this opportunity if we overreact.

But if we turn our overreaction into interaction, then we can share the explicit truth. The Bible isn't afraid to talk about sex in lurid detail. We shouldn't be afraid to either.

So why is it that the church always squirms when we talk about sex? We're so afraid of being "inappropriate" that we avoid talking about the elephant in the room. Meanwhile, Hollywood isn't holding anything back while slinging lies.

Explicit Bible Passages

Perhaps we should start talking about sex the way God designed it . . . as something good!

Sex isn't naughty, it's not inappropriate, and it's not shameful. Sex is an amazing gift that God gives to a man and woman in marriage.

The Bible opens with the story of a naked man in a garden who wants a partner. God sees this and doesn't want Adam to be alone. So what does God do?

Poof. A naked woman!

Then what does God tell Adam? "Go forth and multiply!" How's that for a sexual green light?

God is so awesome!

Why isn't the Bible scared to talk about the subject of sex? The Bible isn't afraid to talk about sex because it's revealed as a gift for us to enjoy in marriage. The Bible tells us the unedited truth throughout its pages. Take Proverbs 5:18–19, for example:

> Let your wife be a fountain of blessing for you.
> Rejoice in the wife of your youth.
> She is a loving deer, a graceful doe.
> Let her breasts satisfy you always.
> May you always be captivated by her love.

I love using this passage to talk with young people about sex for several reasons. First, it's always good to drive students to Scripture, and for some reason, young people always like passages like this one.

Second, this passage is a voice not often heard in the world today—mainly because it's pro-marriage. It talks about marriage not only in a positive light, but also about the passion and intoxication that this kind of relationship brings.

Very romantic.

Third, it doesn't hold back on the specifics; it brings up the fact that a man can enjoy his wife's breasts (and it's not naughty to do so). How often do you hear this in the church? Not often (because people might walk out). But we hear these kinds of details everywhere else in our sexualized world.

Finally, I like using this passage because here the Bible is realistic about the consequences of a husband engaging in sexual activity with other women. The rest of this Proverb goes into more detail about the results of this kind of folly.

This is an amazing passage to go through with young people. It paints a pretty graphic picture of how wonderful it is for a man to enjoy his wife sexually. The passage isn't even afraid to talk about her breasts!

Yes, I realize that passages like this can be a little embarrassing to talk about with our kids. When I read a passage like this, my youngest daughter always interrupts me and says, "Dad, ewwww!"

Let's face it. Sex is an intimate act between a man and woman, so it's okay to feel a little bit awkward when we talk about it. But don't let awkwardness silence you. The Bible isn't silent, so we shouldn't be either. We should discuss it maturely and sensitively.

Sadly, many parents are afraid that having conversations about sex will give their kids ideas and get them thinking about it. These parents are scared of saying *too much*.

Too Much or Too Little?

Think about this for a minute. Are you really afraid of telling your kids too much? Do you really think our kids live in a shoebox? Do you think they've never heard the word *breasts* before?

When it comes to talking about sex with our kids, we can err on the side of giving them *too much information*, or *too little information*. Which side would you prefer to err on?

I've met a lot of parents who, in fear, would rather err on the side of telling them *too little*. I'd love to ask these folks a question. What happens if you actually tell your kids a *little more* unedited truth than they were already exposed to? Is it dangerous to tell them that sex is an amazing gift from God that they can enjoy when they are married?

Do you think if you show a teen or tween this Proverbs Scripture he or she is going to start downloading porn? Do you think that if you use the word *breasts* they are suddenly going to start thinking about breasts all day?

Don't get me wrong. I'm not saying we should throw discernment and wisdom out the window. We don't want to introduce our kids to temptations they've never thought about. That's why it's good to become familiar with media messages our kids are actually listening to. Then if we hear lyrics about oral sex, we can address oral sex, knowing we aren't introducing something new.

And let me just emphasize something: I've *never* met a parent who tried to tell the truth to their kids about sex and ended up introducing their kids to a temptation instead. It just doesn't happen today. The majority of parents think *There's no way my kid knows about oral sex,* when in actuality, their kids have heard other kids talking about it at school, they've heard songs about it, they've seen it inferred in a movie. . . . Parents rarely introduce their kids to temptation while trying to tell them the truth.

So why are many of us so afraid to share too much that we settle for sharing too little?

What if we *do* share too little? What if our kids would really like to know about sex but are too scared to ask? What if they have questions that aren't being answered because we're tiptoeing around the issue? They probably won't raise their hand in youth group or walk into your room before bedtime and say, "*Mom, I'm masturbating every night. I can't stop. It started with the JCPenney catalog and now it's Internet porn. Help!*"

We need to start talking openly and honestly about sex. I'm not trying to give license to flippant use of coarse slang. Far from it! Personally, when I'm talking about sex in a youth group setting or with my own kids, I like to use the word that is the least offensive or "creepy." This can change from crowd to crowd. Some people will tell you to always use the scientific words. Just make sure you know your audience. Some kids will cringe if you use words like *intercourse* or *coitus*.

But definitely don't hesitate to share Scripture like Proverbs 5. Believe it or not, you're going to encounter people who say that it's simply inappropriate to talk about the subject of women's breasts at all. (I hope they never open up their Bible to Song of Songs.) This sort of logic is just bad discernment with no biblical backing. If this were true, then why does the Bible talk about sex in detail time and time again?

The Bible isn't afraid to talk about body parts and sexuality in lurid detail. If you think the Proverbs passage is explicit, then read Genesis 38:8–10 or Ezekiel 23:19–21. You may need to sit down first, though.

Not Ashamed

The fact is plain and simple. The Bible isn't ashamed to talk about good sex the way it was intended, and it's not afraid to denounce sexual immorality just the same (or in the case of the Ezekiel passage above, even use explicit sexual immorality as an analogy to awaken God's people to the kind of adultery they were committing against him). This Proverbs passage talks about how husbands should enjoy their wives' breasts. The key is, these body parts are not something bad. Sex is not naughty. God created this whole process. It's not bad or dirty or shameful.

So often, Christian adults are afraid to talk about "the naughty thing." Satan loves this! The church has unintentionally propagated this lie for years. Our kids have learned that *sex is naughty and we don't talk about it!*

The result?

Our kids sneak around to find answers elsewhere . . . from the people who are talking about it: their friends at school, and in movies, songs, and TV shows . . .

Don't be afraid to tell your kids the truth. Sex is amazing, a gift from God. It's something they'll eventually get to experience when they find the right person and commit to them in marriage.

This isn't naughty . . . *it's just good teaching.*

Talking with our kids about this holistic biblical picture of sex isn't usually accomplished in one conversation. In fact, most experts agree we need to stop thinking of these conversations as "the sex talk." Today's kids don't need one talk. They need continual conversations.

Let's look at how we can create a comfortable climate for these continual conversations in our homes.

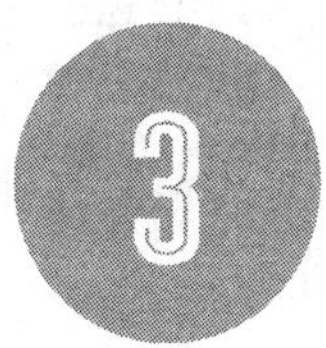

Opening the Doorways of Communication

Creating a comfortable climate for continual conversations

Where do your kids go with their questions about sex?

Think about that one for a moment. At school they hear someone mention something about a sexual act or position. Believe me, it happens more than you think. Or they're watching YouTube, TV, or a movie at their friend's house and one of the characters makes a crude sex joke referencing something your child hasn't heard about before.

What do your kids do with this partial information? Are they curious about the term they just heard?

Gossip spreads about a cheerleader at school. Apparently she drank too much at a party and ended up engaging in some pretty wild activities. The word *anal* is used. Is this a new term for your kids? Will they want to know more?

In a recent article about kids and Internet porn, Martin Daubney shared an eye-opening experience observing sex education consultant Jonny Hunt interact about sex and relationships with a group of people ages thirteen to fourteen. To gain an understanding of what these children knew about sex, Hunt began by asking them each to write an A–Z list of the sexual terms they knew, no matter how explicit. Daubney described the group as children who "had just hit puberty and some were clearly still children: wide-eyed, nervous, with high-pitched voices. Some of the girls were beginning their first forays into makeup. Several wore braces on their teeth. Everybody was smartly turned out in school uniform."

When they posted the list on the board, it was quickly evident that the children's knowledge of porn terms was not only surprisingly extensive, "it superseded that of every adult in the room—including the sex education consultant himself."

"The first word every single boy and girl in the group put on their list was *anal*."

When questioned, every single child in the class of twenty had seen sodomy acted out in porn. Daubney confessed, "I was stunned they even knew about it—I certainly hadn't heard of it at that age—let alone had watched it and as a result may even have wanted to try it."[1] (Which is why we will devote an entire chapter to the subject of pornography—chapter 9.)

If only this was an anomaly.

Been to the grocery store? Just hope your daughter's eyes didn't wander over to that *Cosmopolitan* magazine on the rack that read, "Is anal bleaching safe?" Kristen Wiig joked about it in the popular movie *Bridesmaids* years ago, and *Cosmo* claims, "More and more women are whitening back there."[2] Something that used to be common only with porn stars.

If we ever let our kids out of the house, they most likely have stumbled upon references like this . . . more than we'd like, I'm sure.

Will it make them wonder?

Will they ask their friends?

Will they ask you?

Think about it. Where do they go for answers?

Sadly, the number one place young people go to for answers today is Google.

You can't blame them; it's where we go for everything. How do you fix a leaky faucet? Google it. How do you clean up a raspberry lemonade stain from white carpet? Google it.

Google's a great place to search for how to change your alternator . . . but not always so great for sex advice.

Do you have any idea what our children will discover when they type "anal sex" into the search engine?

How come they don't ask Mom or Dad?

Well . . . *would you have asked your mom or dad?*

As I sit writing this, in the last month I've spoken to twelve- to fourteen-year-olds about sex twice at churches in two different states. Each time a squeaky-voiced middle school boy came up to talk with me afterward, with specific questions, articulate questions . . . *embarrassing questions*. In these situations, which happen more often than you'd think, if I ask, "Have you talked with your mom or dad about this?" I always get the exact same reaction: a laugh, and then a stare clearly communicating, *Are you kidding?*

In author Shaunti Feldhahn's book *For Parents Only*, she asked teenagers about their communication with their parents. Three out of four kids in her survey said they would *like* to share things with their parents—as long as they were sure they wouldn't overreact. In others words, "I'd like to ask Mom this question, but I'm pretty sure she'd flip out."

Think about how it would look in your home.

"Mom, what's anal sex?"

"WHAT! Where did you hear that?! Was it Chris? I knew I should never let you hang out with that boy!"

And we wonder why they go to Google.

The plain truth is, the key to talking to our kids about sex is creating a comfortable climate that cultivates calm and continual conversations. (Nice use of alliteration, huh?) Our kids might be a little more inclined to approach us with these questions if we prove to them that we're not only a good source for truth, but a *safe* source.

What's the key?

I find these four tips help parents create a comfortable climate of continual communication:

Tip #1: Don't Overreact

Or as our kids would say, *"Don't freak out!"*

I know, I know. This is tough. When my youngest daughter was in fifth grade she came home from school, threw her backpack on the couch, and asked, "Dad, what's a blow job?"

My ninth-grade son dropped to the ground in hysterics.

How do you respond to that question?

By God's grace, I was actually calm with my response, probably because I was so excited she felt comfortable enough to ask us those kinds of questions. After twenty years of youth ministry, I have met plenty of young people who know that sex is not a welcome subject in their home.

As calm as possible I asked my daughter, "Well, help me understand the situation so I know better how to answer that."

Yes . . . *I was stalling*!

Helpful hint: When your kids shock you or stump you with a question you don't know how to respond to, stall by asking a question. This will accomplish two things. One, it will buy you time to think. Two, it will give you more context so you know why your kid is asking the question.

That's what I did. I basically said, "Tell me more." It's best to say this not like a parole officer seeking incriminating evidence, but like a psychiatrist gathering information so he can provide better counsel.

She told me she had heard it from a guy named Tyler in her class. We'd heard quite a few stories about this Tyler kid, none of them good.

So I addressed the question the best I could.

"It's an intimate sexual act that two people do, something that married people might really enjoy. Sometimes people who aren't married do it as well, but it's sad, because God really designed intimacy like this for marriage." I did my best to provide an age-appropriate response. I answered her question honestly, providing as much detail as I felt a fifth-grader needed.

Without any hesitation, Ashley dropped another bomb. "So do you and Mom do it?"

Now *I* was trying not to drop on the floor in hysterics. But I finally mustered, "Well, intimate acts like that are really private—things husbands and wives get to enjoy together. If they do them, it's not something they talk about with others. Someday when you get married and you get all huggy and kissy with your husband, you'll really enjoy getting intimate with him, and . . ."

That's as far as I got and she thrust her hand in the air. "Enough. I got it."

These situations aren't easy. It's tough being put on the spot. But if we freak out, they won't put us on the spot anymore, because they won't want to talk to us at all!

Our kids would love to have someone they can trust to go to with tough questions.

Are you that person? Or do you freak out when they bring up distressing stuff?

Remember to do your best to remain calm, buy time with a question or statement like, "Tell me more," and try to convert your overreaction into interaction.

And when you do get the opportunity to interact . . . keep the next tip in mind.

Tip #2: Don't Make Sex "Naughty"

I don't know how it happened. Maybe it's a side effect of our puritanical roots. Possibly it's an attempt to grasp at morality in an overly sexualized culture. Regardless of the cause, many of today's believers in the United States have stained God's gift of sex, making it hush-hush, giving it a stigma.

It's "naughty."

That's what we've learned, so we tend to not talk about the naughty thing too much.

Think about this for a second. Sex is rampant in our culture, it's a huge desire for young boys, it's a huge pressure for young girls . . . *and we don't talk about it!* This breeds ignorance in the Christian community. The one subject kids would really *like* to talk about . . . we hush . . . or only talk about it once for thirty minutes at youth group on Valentine's Day weekend. The rest of the year, we stifle it and hope they don't think about it.

News flash: They're thinking about it frequently. They're hearing about it repeatedly. They're seeing images of it on display daily.

All this focus on sex from society stimulates thoughts and questions . . . thoughts and questions they have to keep suppressed because they don't want to feel naughty.

This creates a negative spiral. When parents see sexual images and hear sexual messages in entertainment media, our response is usually to turn it off or say something negative about it.

"We can't watch that movie, it has sex in it."

What do kids hear? *Sex is naughty.*

"Don't listen to that song, it's about sex."

What do kids hear? *Sex is naughty.*

Is your car naughty? Are you ashamed to have a driver's license? Well, the Centers for Disease Control revealed that automobile accidents are the leading cause of death for U.S. teens.[3] That's no joke! Nothing else kills more of our kids than cars.

So why do we drive cars? Shouldn't we ban all cars since these crashes are taking lives?

I think you get my point. Cars aren't bad, but when people speed, text, drink, fall asleep at the wheel, or drive unsafe in any way . . . people can die.

Similarly, sex isn't bad, but when people go outside of God's design . . . people can literally die. So should we ban God's gift of sex altogether? Should we hush any conversation about it?

Christians need to stop treating sex like it's evil.

Now don't get me wrong, I'm not saying you should let your kids watch porn or stream raunchy music and listen to Lil Wayne bragging about his exploits with his "ladies." (He uses a different word.) Far from it. But let's not confuse sexual perversion with sex.

Sex is amazing!

Sex is God's gift to married couples.

Sex is not only extremely enjoyable, it bonds husband and wife together.

There's nothing bad about sex between a husband and a wife.

Movies, TV shows, websites, music videos, and songs often include sexual content and images because they know people enjoy sex and are curious about it. Sadly, much of the sexual imagery we see and hear in entertainment media isn't God's design. It's about people who indulge in sex outside of marriage. It's about someone who is lusting after someone they're not married to. It's perverting God's original design for sex. It's putting the wonderful private act of sex on display for others to watch, so something beautiful is distorted to be nothing more than lust.

When we encounter perversions of sex, we should point them out as just that.

That's too bad. I really like Jess, and this is a cleverly written TV show, but she just keeps hooking up with guys she meets in bars with no apparent consequences. What do you think really happens when people have casual sex with multiple partners? What are the chances of her contracting an STD or encountering emotional regret?

Some parents might even add:

If this show continues to communicate these lies, we probably shouldn't watch it. I'd hate for you to get the wrong idea about sex. Sex is a great part of the marriage relationship.

Contrast that to if parents erupted, "Jess is a whore from the house of Jezebel. We won't be watching any of this perversion in this house!"

In other words, "Sex is what naughty people do."

Message received loud and clear.

I'm guessing that most of you aren't exploding into tirades about whores or Jezebel. But we might want to reflect on what messages we do communicate about sex.

"I hate all the sex in these shows. We aren't going to watch that filth!"

"We aren't going to listen to songs with those dirty sexual lyrics."

What do our kids hear? Hate . . . sex . . . filth . . . dirty. Bottom line: sex is naughty.

Is it too much of a stretch to consider our kids might even conclude:

When I'm having these sexual thoughts that I struggle with . . . I'm naughty. I better not say anything because I know how Mom and Dad will react.

Learn to be more specific in your objection to inappropriate sexual content. Calmly and casually communicate, "Wow, these music videos are showing a lot of women in provocative situations. What do you think will happen if men frequently watch women in videos like this instead of enjoying their own wives? What does the Bible call that?" (Later in the book we're going to provide examples of more conversations where you can talk with your kids about "fleeing" these kinds of temptations, and what that actually looks like.)

I know this can be difficult at times. Sex is also something people do in private and can be embarrassing to talk about. Married couples don't typically open up family dinner conversation with, "Last night your mother and I were . . ." And I'm not suggesting you do.

Let's just be careful not to distort this amazing gift from God. Don't confuse your kids by making all sex sound naughty. Instead, help your kids understand what good sex is—between a husband and wife. Then they'll be able to spot counterfeits on their own. Help them recognize when sex is being exploited and used as mere "eye candy." Teach them to "flee" visuals that cause them to lust.

As parents, it's our job to be advocates of the truth. The world will constantly put sex on display and communicate, *"Have sex whenever it feels right!"* Young people who believe that will end up gravely disappointed in the long run. So we need to be a voice of truth. A big part of that is not misrepresenting sex as something naughty.

Today's young people are much more likely to talk with someone who isn't always angry and ranting about sexual immorality.

Create a climate that cultivates communication about this awesome gift God has given us. It's not naughty, and it's not something we should hush.

In fact, we should keep our eyes open for opportunities to engage in these kinds of conversations.

Tip #3: Keep Your Eyes Open for Natural Springboards

Life is full of little reminders about sex and our sexuality. Use these opportunities to dialogue.

When our kids are young, many of these opportunities will arise when they ask questions. Most children are full of questions.

"Why does my penis get big sometimes?"

"Why do girls have vaginas and boys have penises?"

"What are nipples for?"

Don't hush these questions; just try your best to answer them calmly. Be honest but brief. No need to go on and on. If you don't know what to say right away, use the trick of asking a question in response to buy yourself some time.

"That's a good question. What do you think nipples are for?"

This might only buy you a second or two if they answer, "I don't know." At this point, you just have to do your best to answer calmly and scientifically. (We'll look at more of these tough questions and answers in chapter 12.)

Don't try to cover all of human sexuality in one talk. Spread it out over numerous little conversations. If your kids are like mine were, they'll ask questions frequently.

It's funny, but parents are often scared to answer their kids' questions. They're afraid their kids will grow up too soon if they give them information about sexuality.

I asked my friend Marv Penner about this last month when we ate breakfast together at a youth convention where we both spoke. Marv is the director of the Canadian Centre of Adolescent

Research. He has more than thirty years in the field, and is the author of *The Youth Worker's Guide to Parent Ministry* and *Help! My Kids Are Hurting*.

I asked Marv, "Parents always ask me, 'What answer do I give my eight-year-old if they ask questions about sex?'"

Marv didn't even blink. He just took a bite of his yogurt and said, "Answer whatever your kids are asking!"

Laughing, I asked, "Yeah, but is there a chance parents might mess it up?"

"Sure," Marv explained, "if they assume that giving kids a knowledge of biology gives them a knowledge of morality."

That's why it's good to not just teach body parts, but include the big picture of how God created us. My friend Jim Burns wrote two books I recommend. *God Made Your Body* is a fully illustrated book where children ages three to five will learn that boys' and girls' bodies are different—and "those differences mean boys and girls can grow up to become daddies and mommies." *How God Makes Babies* helps children ages six to nine understand that "God created males and females differently and with a purpose."

Books like these can help us be proactive about teaching body parts, sexuality, and God's design.

We need to make sure to have these discussions before our kids hit puberty. Today, puberty typically begins between eight and thirteen for girls, and nine and fifteen for boys. I've known girls who found out about menstruation the hard way—one day they found blood in their Hello Kitty panties. My daughter had a friend at school whose parents never talked with her about sexuality or the changes in a girl's body. She went to the bathroom in the middle of class and discovered blood in her underwear.

To quote my daughter, "She went ballistic!"

Parents can't ignore these natural landmarks in their kids' lives. In fact, parents need to be proactively talking about some of these issues rather than reactively trying to explain to their hysterical daughter why her vagina is bleeding.

If a parent has frequent conversations with her daughter about her body, explaining her cycle, menstruation, breast growth, and pubic hair growth, then these changes won't come as a surprise. And when some of these body changes do happen, use them as natural springboards to talk about sexuality.

Talks about *sexuality* will open doors to conversations about *sex*. *Sexuality* involves conversations about body parts, growth, and the differences between boys and girls. *Sex* is the act of making love, which can be for pleasure and reproduction. Talks about sexuality don't always necessitate talking about sex.

When your boy is four and five, you might read an illustrated book to him about the human body. When he's six and seven, you might end up answering some deeper questions about erections and images he notices. By the time he hits double digits, he might even stop asking questions. That's when you might need to be the one who initiates these conversations. One way to do that is . . .

Tip #4: Ask, Listen . . . Repeat

Look for opportunities to ask well-placed questions.

Let's be honest. Even in homes where parents rarely overreact and where the subject of sex isn't hush-hush, the topic still can be awkward for everyone. We are talking about something very intimate, and as wonderful as sex is, it's an activity two people do in private.

So don't expect your twelve-year-old son to walk right up to you and say, "Mom, I feel horny all the time. In fact, I have trouble even walking through the mall without lustful thoughts popping into my head when I pass most store windows. Oh . . . and I masturbate daily."

Some kids will be this bold—but very few. This is embarrassing subject matter.

That is why many parents avoid the discussions completely. They figure that if their kids need something, they'll ask.

Sadly, many kids never do.

We can help our kids engage in meaningful conversations about sex by keeping our eyes open for opportunities to ask well-placed questions. Like when a dad notices his twelve-year-old son is beginning to notice pictures of women on the front of magazine covers at the grocery store.

"It seems like these magazines always have a pretty girl on the front of them, huh?"

It's a harmless question, it's not accusatory, and it actually doesn't even require a long answer. It's mere fishing to see how your son will respond. If he says, "Yuck. Where are the video game magazines?" he might not be interested in girls yet . . . or he could be covering up any embarrassment. Use relaxed, non-confronting questions to fish some more.

If your son agrees with your question and says, "Yeah, and they are always wearing small bikinis," then you have an open door to a conversation.

"Do many girls at your school wear bikinis at the end-of-the-year party at the water park? . . . Are any of them pretty?"

Don't worry. You aren't leading your kid down a path of lust; you're just letting him know it's okay to talk to you about his feelings, including how he feels about the opposite sex.

If your son's face lights up and he acknowledges his interest in girls, then you might have found an open door to talk about how God made us.

"God made women pretty like that, and someday you might find a woman you are really attracted to—not just her looks, but everything about her. Have you ever felt that way about a girl?"

Give a little bit of information, and then ask a question to check in and see if he is tracking with you. That might lead you to a conversation about a girl he likes. Maybe you'll have a chance to share a little more.

"Someday you'll probably even fall in love with a woman and marry her. Marriage is cool, because married people commit to become not only best friends, but to love each other intimately. Hugs, kisses . . . and much more. What do you think of that?"

Again, a little more information, followed by a question.

No need to rush into the full-scale explanation of intercourse every time. Remember, we don't need to have just one "sex talk." Today's kids need hundreds.

When kids are younger, it's okay to say things like "married people hug, kiss, and much more." One day, your kid will ask you, "What do you mean more?" That's a great cue that they're ready to hear a little more about God's design. If you don't know exactly how much they have already heard about sex, just ask them when the subject arises. Whenever they are introduced to their first sex education class at school—usually around fourth or fifth grade, ask them, "What did you learn today?"

Remember, school often will teach them the biology but not the morality. Kids might learn how the body works, but they typically won't hear the answers to specific questions like, *When is it okay to have sex? How do I know how far I should go with my boyfriend or girlfriend?* Or even, *Where do I look to find the truth about these issues?* Parents can help their kids discover the truth to these common questions.

I'll outline what some of these conversations look like in the next few chapters, but you can also use resources written directly to your teens and tweens, like my book *Sex Matters*, which clearly presents God's design for sex, answering questions like "Should I wait?" and "How far is too far?" It even has discussion questions at the end of each chapter. Books like this can be great ways to discuss biblical truth with your kids.

Create a comfortable climate that cultivates continued conversations. Not one sex talk, but an ongoing dialogue.

You can keep using this approach, and if your kid is putting up huge walls and changing the subject, then back off. Try again another time.

Don't let the content scare you off. My friend Marv, whom I quoted earlier in this chapter, said, "Talking with your kids about sex has little to do with the content but everything to do with the quality of the relationship." I can't agree more. Don't worry about being eloquent or giving the perfect presentation. Just love your kids and be there for them. Keep your eyes open for these opportunities and make them feel noticed and heard.

Questions help us with the listening part. They keep us in check to make sure that we don't lecture blindly. Questions help us move from monologue to dialogue.

Note the word *dialogue*.

Most homes probably have a little too many *monologues*, where Dad or Mom is lecturing. I know I could have been blamed for this many times in my home. Mere lectures often miss the mark, because they don't stop and take the pulse of the listener.

Parents should try a little more listening than lecturing. *Dialogue* is waaaaaaaaay more effective than monologue.

When it comes to talking about sex, look for open doors and ask a question. If the time is right, provide a little bit of information followed by a question. Question, info, question . . .

I gave the example of a dad talking with his son. This works with our daughters too.

"Why do you think she's dressed like that in most of her music videos?"

"I don't know." (A common answer.)

"What do you think most guys are thinking when they see her dressed like that?"

"They probably like it."

"So do you think we should all dress like that, so guys will like us?"

"No."

"Why not?"

The conversation could take a million turns. Fish with a question, provide a little information, followed by another question. (We'll look more at these kinds of conversations with our daughters in chapter 6.)

The more we have these conversations, the easier it will be for our kids to talk with us. Give them opportunities to test the waters. Prove you won't freak out. Make them feel unconditionally loved and unquestionably accepted, not naughty, when they have sexual thoughts or desires. And demonstrate that you are easy to talk to because you listen and provide relevant information.

Become a safe voice in your kids' lives, and next time they have a question about sex . . . *maybe they'll come to you instead of Google.*

The Most Enjoyable Sex

Answering the biggest question young people ask: "Why wait?"

Why wait?

It's the question young people are thinking about *but not asking.*

The question is probably a little more emphatic than that for some. Many young people today are thinking:

> *People engage in casual sexual encounters in every TV show I watch and in every movie I enjoy. Whenever I am online, distracting pictures bombard me, begging me to click and see more, and honestly, I'm curious. Kids at school talk about sex, and my favorite songs obsess about it. Let's be real . . . everybody seems to think the idea of waiting is absurd! In fact, people are mocked for thinking this way.*
>
> *But my mom and dad tell me the Bible says to wait. Can I believe the Bible?*
>
> *Give me just one compelling reason to wait! And don't try to scare me with teen pregnancy, because there are literally hundreds*

of kids at my school having sex, and none of them . . . seriously, not one . . . are pregnant.

There it is. The burden of proof is on us. We're in the minority if we think sex is a gift to be enjoyed between married couples. Our kids are hearing the opposite message every day.

Many of them are sorting it out in their minds, weighing the evidence on both sides, especially as they grow into their later high school years. "Should I really wait until marriage?"

If you haven't answered this question, then most likely your kids are seeking these answers on their own. In fact, some have already made their decision. In the U.S., about one-third of high school freshmen have already had sexual intercourse, precisely 32 percent of boys and 28.1 percent of girls. The number goes up each year. By the time U.S. students are in their senior year of high school, 64 percent of them have already had sexual intercourse.[1]

What will your kids decide?

Have you provided a compelling answer to their question, "Should I wait?"

In chapter 1 we were reminded of the many loud voices answering that question for our kids. Most of those voices are saying, *"Don't wait. If it feels right, do it."*

How can we combat these messages?

What do these conversations look like?

Entertainment media likes to joke about parental attempts to caution their kids about casual sex. I can't help but think of the pilot episode of the cult classic Judd Apatow TV show *Freaks and Geeks*, starring Seth Rogen, James Franco, Jason Segel, and others. Sam is eating a family meal and his dad awkwardly announces:

Harold: You know, there was a girl in our school . . . and she had premarital sex. Know what she did on her graduation day? Died! Of a heroin overdose!

Sam: Dad? Are any of your friends alive?

Harold: The smart ones.

Is that all we have to offer? Fear tactics? False fears, at that?

The fact is, *truth* is on our side. And in a world full of explicit lies, our kids need to hear the explicit truth.

When I was a kid, I heard plenty of people tell me, "Wait until marriage for sex." But for me, *Why?* was huge. I wanted to know all the details so I could make my *own* decision. I don't think I'm the only one.

Most young people aren't going to be convinced with "because the Bible says so." Some will want to see those passages for themselves. *Are they clear? Are you sure you didn't interpret them wrong?*

Some kids won't even consider the Bible as a valid source. *Is there other evidence that sex is worth the wait? Or are Christians just clinging to an outdated book?*

These are good questions. Interestingly enough, whether young people care about the Bible or not, both research and common sense actually support what the Bible communicates clearly. In fact, I think the more our kids look at God's amazing gift of sex, the more they're going to see that God isn't trying to keep anything from them; he just wants a better life for them.

Let's take a look at three compelling reasons why waiting is wise. We'll answer this biblically, scientifically, and logically.

1. The Biblical Answer

Can you guess the number one reason young people gave for waiting for sex?

I would probably guess *fear of STDs* or *teen pregnancy.*

Nope and nope.

The Centers for Disease Control (CDC) asked young people who abstained why they waited, and the number one reason was . . .

God.

The survey was the National Survey of Family Growth (NSFG), and it revealed the number one reason teenagers provided for not having sex was that it was "against religion or morals." Forty-one percent of females and 31 percent of males between the ages of fifteen and nineteen claimed religion or morals as the reason they were waiting. The second and third reasons for abstaining were the fear of getting pregnant and "haven't found the right person yet."[2]

Fear of STDs wasn't even in the top three.

I've been speaking to young people for over twenty years, and I can honestly say that the most radical positive life changes I have witnessed have been as a result of a kid's faith.

Faith is a powerful motivator.

But let's not be foolish and celebrate that a mere third of those teenagers are actually waiting for sex because of their convictions. Seriously? Only a third? Why not the other two-thirds?

Sadly, many young people today aren't taught the truth about God's plan for sex. Sure, they might have heard, "Don't have sex," or sadly, "Sex is bad." But I have met very few young people who can actually articulate what the Bible says about sex.

Can your kids tell you what the Bible says?

Don't wait for their youth pastor or Sunday school teacher to tell them. As parents, it's our job to let them know God's design is best.

Why should we wait until marriage to have sex?

That's the big question we're seeking to answer here. And the Bible provides a great answer.

God Created Sex for Us to Enjoy in Marriage for Life

In short, God's design is ultimately the most enjoyable.

Does that claim surprise you?

When many of us think of the Bible, we think of the "Thou shalt not" passages. Perhaps we should take a peek at what the Bible is telling us to enjoy instead.

Enjoy

Explain to your kids that God's design for sex is evident all through the Bible. Start from the beginning . . . *the very beginning* . . . like the book of Genesis. I mentioned this passage before, but let's look a little deeper this time.

God made a guy named Adam. As Adam walked around and looked at all the animals, he thought, "I like animals and all, but I sure would like a companion I could relate to more."

God noticed this. In Genesis 2:18, God said, "It is not good for the man to be alone."

So while Adam was sleeping, God made him a wife. Adam wakes up, sees this beautiful naked woman, and literally says, "At last!"

> "At last!" the man exclaimed.
> "This one is bone from my bone,
> and flesh from my flesh!
> She will be called 'woman,'
> because she was taken from 'man.'"
> This explains why a man leaves his father and mother
> and is joined to his wife, and the two are united into one.
> Now the man and his wife were both naked, but they felt no shame.
>
> Genesis 2:23–25

Once God made them both, he then told them, "Be fruitful and multiply" (Genesis 1:28).

My guess is that God probably didn't need to convince them to do this.

Some people miss God's awesome gift of sexual enjoyment here because they assume that God's command to "be fruitful and multiply" just meant "have babies." But God's creation was so much more than this. Why did God give both man and woman pleasure centers on their genitals? Think about that for a second. Do you know that the woman's clitoris has no purpose whatsoever other than to provide sexual pleasure? The pleasure centers on the head of the penis are the same way. God gave us the awesome gift of sex for us to *enjoy.*

Sex isn't naughty. In fact, God is a big advocate for sex within marriage. Take that Proverbs 5 passage (which we've already explored), for example:

> Let your wife be a fountain of blessing for you.
> Rejoice in the wife of your youth.

She is a loving deer, a graceful doe.
Let her breasts satisfy you always.
May you always be captivated by her love.
Proverbs 5:18–19

Many young people don't even know the Bible talks like this. But the plain, unedited truth is that God wants a husband to *enjoy* his wife's breasts, and as I mentioned before, the Bible isn't afraid to say that explicitly.

Long-term Fulfillment

Sex is very pleasurable. Just looking at his wife's body can be a stimulating experience for a husband. God made it that way. But let me be clear. God's creation of sexual enjoyment goes well beyond immediate pleasure. God actually also provides a long-term fulfillment for two people when they join together as one (Genesis 2:25) and live as partners for life.

Sex is a big part of this union as "one flesh." It's a special gift created for married couples to share uniquely, and their relationship actually becomes more connected the more the two of them are intimate with each other.

The human body releases a powerful hormone called oxytocin when you hug or kiss someone you really care about. This hormone, often called the bonding hormone or cuddle hormone, is stimulated big-time during sex. It actually deepens the feelings of attachment each time a couple has sex. In one study, men were given oxytocin while they looked at pictures of women—including complete strangers, women they were acquainted with, and women they were in love with. The pleasure and desire regions of their brains lit up at the mere sight of the women they loved.[3]

This is why the pain of a breakup is so great. Think of the thousands of songs written about this kind of hurt. The more we bond with someone and share the most intimate part of ourselves, the more it rips us apart when we separate.

It's almost as if the guy behind the design of all this didn't want us to make that sexual connection unless we meant to stay together, eh?

Marriage

But some people try to get the sexual enjoyment without having to commit to the obligation of marriage.

It makes sense. People like the immediate pleasure sex provides—so much so that they wonder if they can enjoy that quick thrill with lots of partners. They might see marriage as a hassle, not a long-term fulfillment, so they seek the pleasure of a one-night stand or even sex with a prostitute.

God knew people would do this, so he addressed this explicitly in Scripture. Take the next few verses in the Proverbs passage we just read. Right after telling a husband to enjoy his wife's breasts, God gives this warning:

> Why be captivated, my son, by an immoral woman,
>   or fondle the breasts of a promiscuous woman?
> For the Lord sees clearly what a man does,
>   examining every path he takes.
> An evil man is held captive by his own sins;
>   they are ropes that catch and hold him.
> He will die for lack of self-control;
>   he will be lost because of his great foolishness.
>
> Proverbs 5:20–24

In other words, *I created sex for you to enjoy in marriage. In marriage, you can even enjoy the feeling you get when you see and touch your wife's breasts. But that enjoyment is reserved for marriage. Don't enjoy other women's breasts. This temptation will ensnare you and capture you until eventually you will face dire consequences for your "great foolishness."*

Talk with your kids about this passage and some common ways people become "ensnared" by these temptations today. For example, pornography offers a chance for men to be captivated by the breasts of many women; but this passage reveals that it will take us captive and hurt our relationship with our wives and with God.

But let your daughters know this verse isn't just for guys; it applies to females too. God designed sex for both men and women to enjoy in marriage. He goes on to tell us this explicitly throughout the Bible. God gives warnings about sex to married people, single people, and even people who think it might be okay to just think about sex. These warnings are the "Thou shalt not" passages.

What About Sex With People Other Than My Spouse?

Sadly, people often try to do things their own way rather than the way God intended. They think, *Sex is fun, so I'll have it with others as well, not just my spouse.* We see numerous examples of people trying this all through the Bible, even in the first book: Judah (Genesis 38), the people of Sodom and Gomorrah (Genesis 19), and many of the Israelites.

So God warned them in the Ten Commandments, "You must not commit adultery" (Exodus 20:14).

That's pretty clear. Don't have sex outside of marriage.

Again, this isn't because sex was bad or because God wanted to deny their fun. Quite the contrary. He actually created an amazing plan where one man and one woman could join together in a unique bond for the rest of their lives, committed to each other and enjoying the pleasure of sexual intimacy, something the two of them would share exclusively.

What About Sex If I'm Not Married Yet?

Some kids might ask, "Well, I'm not married. Isn't it okay to have sex, because I won't be cheating my spouse . . . since I don't have a spouse?"

First, you have to question the logic there. Just because your child doesn't have a husband or wife yet doesn't mean that they should go bonding with a bunch of other people now. Think of what we know so far about this process. God wants us to enjoy sex with one person for life. That doesn't license us to sleep with a bunch of people before we're married. Everything we do before marriage will be carried into the marriage relationship.

Just in case you missed that logic, the apostle Paul addresses this throughout the New Testament, like this passage: "Run from sexual sin! No other sin so clearly affects the body as this one does. For sexual immorality is a sin against your own body" (1 Corinthians 6:18).

English translations of the Bible will use a variety of different terms here that all mean the same thing: *sexual sin, sexual immorality*, or *fornication*. The Greek words in these "sexual immorality" passages are always *porneia* or *pornos*, which, as the dad from *My Big Fat Greek Wedding* would say, are the root words for the English words *pornography* or *pornographic*. If your pastor looks it up in his Greek dictionary, it will say something like, "the surrendering of sexual purity; promiscuity of any or every type." I like to define it as *the voluntary sex of an unmarried person*.

In other words, run from any temptations to have sex with someone if you're not married to them. Paul uses this term again in Ephesians 5:3: "Let there be no sexual immorality, impurity, or greed among you. Such sins have no place among God's people."

I like the way the New International Version of the Bible words it: "There must not be even a hint of sexual immorality" among you. It's pretty clear. Don't have sex outside of the marriage relationship.

And just in case we've missed either of these categories, Hebrews 13:4 addresses both adulterers and fornicators: "Marriage should be honored by all, and the marriage bed kept pure, for God will judge the adulterer and all the sexually immoral" (NIV).

It seems pretty crystal clear, right?

What About Just Thinking About Sex?

Some people still try to find a loophole. Maybe porn is okay, right? Because then we aren't actually having sex with anyone else. We're just sort of . . . *pretending to have sex in our minds!*

During the time Jesus was walking around earth, he encountered some people like this. They were thinking, *"So as long as I don't have sex, it's okay. I'll just think about it!"*

Jesus himself decided to address this, calling it "lust," and labeling it just as bad as adultery.

> You have heard the commandment that says, "You must not commit adultery." But I say, anyone who even looks at a woman with lust has already committed adultery with her in his heart. So if your eye—even your good eye—causes you to lust, gouge it out and throw

> it away. It is better for you to lose one part of your body than for your whole body to be thrown into hell.
>
> Matthew 5:27–29

Jesus wasn't pulling any punches here.

If you're thinking about it, you're no better than someone who is doing it.

And if you have any doubts about how serious Jesus was about this, just read that part about plucking your eye out again.

God's way makes a lot of sense. In fact, so much sense that research reveals the biblical advice to be pretty smart.

2. The Scientific Answer

I spend quite a bit of time researching youth culture, attitudes, trends, and teen health. In any given week, I'll probably read a dozen articles and a handful of scientific studies about teenagers. In fact, you can see these studies shared on my website for parents, TheSource4Parents.com, where I have a section titled, "Articles Jonathan has read this week."

In the last two decades I've paid particularly close attention to any studies about teen and adult sexuality, sexual satisfaction, and STDs. I speak to teenagers frequently, and I always want to have the most current information.

In writing this book I dove headfirst into a pile of recent studies from different perspectives. After reading through countless reports, I couldn't help but notice a common assertion:

Monogamy Is More Enjoyable

Monogamy literally means "one partner." I am tempted to use the word *marriage* here, but the word *monogamy* doesn't always mean marriage. In today's world, it can now also mean cohabitating couples who are "committed" to each other.

I'll leave it up to you to decide what you think the word *committed* truly means. Because when couples live together, they aren't committed enough to tie the knot in marriage, but they are saying, "I choose you . . . *for now*."

That's the thing about today's "monogamous" relationships outside of marriage. They don't often stay true to the "mono" part of monogamy. So when an unmarried "monogamous" man breaks it off with his partner and then begins living with a new woman, officially that is called "serial monogamy," which is defined as when individuals engage in sequential monogamous pairings, but always one at a time. True monogamy is *one partner for life*. (Dare I say "marriage"?)

Research not only reveals the benefits of true monogamy, but also how much better *one partner for life* is compared to those with multiple partners past (serial monogamy) and multiple partners present (known as polygamy or polyamory) or promiscuity (sleeping with whoever I want whenever I want).

Don't let all these terms confuse you. The bottom line is this: Most research points to the fact that sex is best saved for the intimacy of a true monogamous relationship, *one person for life*. Now that's a good reason to save sex for marriage that we can share with our kids!

Here's a peek at some of the research on the subject.

A few years ago, two sociologists did some research on the subject and wrote an entire book about it, *Premarital Sex in America*. Their study looked at the sexual behaviors of contemporary young adults, and their findings weren't surprising.

As they compared monogamous couples to individuals who were promiscuous, they started to notice patterns. They discovered a significant correlation between the following:

- sexual restraint and emotional well-being
- monogamy and happiness
- promiscuity and depression

In fact, the happiest women they studied "were those with a current sexual partner and only one or two partners in their lifetime." And sadly, "a young woman's likelihood of depression rose steadily as her number of partners climbed and the present stability of her sex life diminished."[4] In other words, the more a woman slept around, the more depressed she became and her sex life grew worse.

Sexual Satisfaction

This research isn't unique. The more you look at the research, the more you'll discover people reported greater sexual satisfaction in monogamous relationships. In fact, this is nothing new.

Let's take a step back a few decades. In the early nineties, a group of social scientists wrote a 718-page monograph reporting the sexual habits of a large cross section of Americans. Several factors came as a surprise to many.

First, the report found there was more emotional satisfaction and physical pleasure for those in a monogamous relationship than for those who had sexual relations with one or more other partners within the past twelve months. In fact, in a sample of 868 women located in fifteen states, the women with many partners expressed the least sexual satisfaction. The more people they slept with, the less happy they were with sex.[5]

Second, the report found a direct correlation between "religious belief" and sexual pleasure. In fact, the study found that the people who have the most sex, experience the best sex, and are the happiest with their sex lives are monogamous, married, religious people. The religious people actually reported more orgasms:

> Women without religious affiliation were the least likely to report always having an orgasm with their primary partner—only one in five. . . . Protestant women who reported always having an orgasm was the highest, at nearly one-third. In general, having a religious affiliation was associated with higher rates of orgasm for women (27 percent of both Catholic and Type I Protestants reported always having an orgasm with their primary partner.)[6]

The authors couldn't help but conclude, "Religion may be independently associated with rates of orgasm."[7]

Whodathunkit?

This wasn't the first study to find the correlation between religion and sexual satisfaction. In fact, one of the largest studies ever attempted found the same thing. *Redbook* magazine surveyed over 100,000 women in the early seventies. They found monogamous women to be more sexually satisfied; furthermore, they discovered "a positive religious approach to sexual pleasure, which links sex and marital fulfillment, is likely to have a considerable effect on women for whom religious authority still serves as a sanctioning force in life."[8]

It didn't matter if the reports were from last year or the last century, I kept reading the same thing—monogamous couples using terms like *sexual satisfaction* and *happiness*. In fact, some use the word *happiness* in the title of their studies, like a recent report by two economists entitled *Money, Sex, and Happiness*. This paper even used the word *marriage*, labeling those in monogamous, faithful marriages the happiest. They found those who cheated on their spouses "less happy" and those who paid for sex "much less happy" than others.[9]

But let's be honest. Are all the reports saying this? Even the recent ones? Because if you're like me, you've stood in line at the grocery store and seen titles of articles on the magazine racks like, "How an Affair Will Boost Your Marriage."

Do these studies advocating promiscuity hold any water? Are people who have affairs happier in the long run?

To answer that question, let's look at this word we keep seeing over and over again: *happiness*.

Defining Happiness

Most of the reports above use words like *happiness* or *sexual satisfaction*. What does that really mean?

Mark White, PhD, offers some good insight into perceived happiness in a recent *Psychology Today* article. He starts off the article declaring, "It doesn't take much to see that monogamy and promiscuity can each give a person happiness, albeit likely two different kinds."

In other words, Dr. White is saying that both monogamy and promiscuity can make someone "happy." But each produces a different kind of happy.

When I show teenagers research like this, I simply tell them to take a look at what he discovered and determine which kind of "happiness" they want.

Promiscuity—The Thrill of the Moment

Promiscuity, or "nonmonogamy" as he calls it, "brings the excitement of variety, the thrill of the unknown, and the pure physical bliss of sex, untethered by any emotional attachment or anxiety."

Monogamy—Longer-Lasting Fulfillment

On the other hand, monogamy provides "a deeper, longer-lasting, and more fulfilling type of happiness that enhances any other aspects of one's life."

I can't say I disagree with his premise. It's almost like he's saying, "Sin is fun for the moment." His observation basically surmises that if we go around having sex with anyone we want, we're going to experience the "bliss" and pleasure that sex brings, without the hassle of emotional attachment, for those who find it a hassle. We'd be fools to deny the "temporary" and quick thrill of sin. If sin wasn't fun, we probably wouldn't do it. Sin can be fun . . . *for the moment*.

It's the consequences that hurt.

White says, "The ideal would be to find the more hedonic, animalistic pleasure with his or her spouse or partner instead of looking for it outside the marriage or relationship." I can't help but agree!

Ask your teenagers what they are looking for: the quick thrill or, to use White's words, the "longer-lasting and more fulfilling type of happiness"?[10]

In the last decade, one of the most popular shows among twelve- to seventeen-year-olds was *Jersey Shore*. In this show, young adults basically lived life doing whatever they wanted: drinking, sleeping around, clubbing, and partying. What did you see if you watched that show? Two things: *sex* and *drama*. Arguing, backbiting, jealousy, fighting, name-calling, outbursts of anger, etc. No one would deny it.

It's funny how life turns out when we try to do it our own way instead of God's way.

People in search of "happiness" and "enjoyment" often look for it in the wrong places.

God created us to enjoy sex in a relationship where we'll never need to worry about disease, never need to compare with others, and never feel guilty afterward. Those who have sex in marriage enjoy a longer-lasting, more fulfilled happiness and are more satisfied with sexual intimacy with their spouse.

God wants us to experience the most enjoyable sex, and research reveals that's most commonly found in the context of marriage.

But let's look at God's design another way. . . .

3. The Logical Answer

God's design just makes sense.

Whenever I'm speaking to kids I always tell them, "Close your eyes and picture this world."

Then I help them visualize a picture of this world exactly how you see it every day . . . with one small exception: Everyone believes God's plan for sex and marriage.

I paint the picture just like this:

I want you to picture this world for a minute. Picture it exactly how you see it every day. Picture the things you find beautiful and the things you enjoy, what makes you laugh, what makes you smile. But let's be realistic. Let's also recognize some of the pain in this world: wars, world hunger, sickness, brutality, death . . . the list goes on. This is the world we live in.

Now I want you to make one small adjustment to this image, one little tweak to change your picture. Just imagine the world exactly like it is now . . . but with one exception: Everyone in the entire world believes God's plan for sex and marriage and stays true to their one spouse for life.

The world still has suicide, crime, high school dropouts, and all other kinds of pain and hurt. If you ride your bike to the grocery store and leave it out front unlocked, it will be gone within five minutes because people steal things in this world.

But even with all this pain and hurt, every single person believes God's plan to wait until sex for marriage, and no one performs any sexual activity outside of the marriage relationship. No one lusts after one another, and once they get married, they love each other and stay committed to their spouses, enjoying a sexual intimacy with just the two of them for the rest of their lives.

Picture this world:

- *For starters, in this world, Dad doesn't trade in his wife for a younger version.*
- *This is a world with no dads cheating on moms, or moms cheating on dads.*
- *There are no painful family splits because couples actually love each other and stay committed to each other in this world.*
- *This is a world with no pornography, because no one is lusting and no one would pose for sexual pictures for that purpose.*
- *This is a world with no prostitution, because sex is only for marriage.*
- *This is a world with no pedophiles, no molestation, and no sexual abuse of any kind, because again, sex is only between a husband and wife in the intimacy of marriage.*
- *This world doesn't have any "Who's Your Daddy?" reality TV shows, and probably has no idea who a Kardashian is.*
- *This is a world with no STDs. No AIDS would be transmitted sexually from partner to partner, no gonorrhea, no herpes, no syphilis.*
- *This is a world with no chlamydia, the asymptomatic STD that often leads to pelvic inflammatory disease and eventually infertility problems in women.*
- *This is a world with no HPV, the human papillomavirus, which is the leading cause of cervical cancer in women.*[11]

- *This is a world with very few abortions, whereas in the "real world," 83 percent of abortions are performed on women who are not married.*[12]
- *This is a world with no rape.*
- *This is a world with no sex slavery.*

. . . the list goes on. All this if people just trusted God in this one area of their lives. Imagine if they trusted him in everything.

Let me ask you . . . Does God's way sound so bad?

Worth the Wait

Sex is worth the wait.

I got married at twenty years old. I've now been married over twenty years. It's weird looking back. . . . I actually have lived more years married than I have single.

I can't even imagine being on my own anymore.

I constantly tell my kids:

> When I was young, it seemed like I was going to have to wait forever to get married. That handful of years seemed to move by so slow. But after you have been married for twenty years, the few years before you were married truly seem like nothing.
>
> You have a whole lifetime to have lots of great sex, and saving yourself for marriage will only make that lifetime of sex better.
>
> If you get married, and you both serve each other like the Bible asserts, you will also be having more sex than your "promiscuous" friends . . . a lot more sex. In addition, you will also be having better sex—the best sex, actually.
>
> The answer is simply *discipline*. Your discipline now is a gift to your future spouse. All you are doing is trading a few years of *discipline* for a lifetime of *awesome* connecting in ways you probably can't even imagine yet.
>
> Someday, like Adam, you will realize that the greatest thing God ever invented is lying right next to you in your marriage bed. And you get to enjoy connecting with that person, in so many exciting ways, for the rest of your life.

My kids know I feel this way. God's gift of marriage is such an amazing blessing. My wife, Lori, and I are friends, we're kayaking buddies, we run together, we eat wings at Buffalo Wild Wings together and also the fancy fish place she likes . . .

. . . and we're lovers.

God's plan for sex is so amazing!

God's way is the best way. When we try to do it our own way, we bring consequences on ourselves: physical consequences, emotional consequences, and spiritual consequences. If we look at the outcome of our choices, it's even more evident that God's way is best.

God wants us to enjoy sex with the person we marry forever. He doesn't want us to have a sneak preview. It's wrong and it robs us of that special gift. God has given us the gift of sex to enjoy in marriage.

Talk with your kids about that gift. And treasure that gift . . . *the way God intended it.*

How Far?

Answering the biggest question young Christians ask: "How far can I go?"

During high school I had a serious girlfriend. We dated for almost a year and we spent every possible moment together. We started as friends, but that quickly escalated to something more.

I waited about a month to kiss her for the first time. I won't bore you with the details, but within a few months, it wasn't uncommon for our time together to include long make-out sessions.

Something began happening. The more time we spent making out, the more difficult it was to stop it from going further.

You probably know exactly what I'm talking about.

It's almost as if God's design is that once you start passionately kissing . . . *you want to keep going!*

This is where the inevitable question is asked:

How far can we go?

It's the biggest question Christians in relationships are forced to wrestle with almost every day.

Some couples never discuss it. This is the surest way to fail. *Just hope it doesn't progress.* Any couple who has dated for any length of time and gets alone will quickly discover that kissing leads to passionate embraces, which evolve to groping . . . until soon it takes a dad with a shotgun to stop things from progressing further!

Those couples who do address the question usually are searching for a line. If they've read the Bible at all and studied some of the verses we've already addressed in this book, they know that sex is for marriage. But what is sex? Sex is just intercourse, right?

So the search for "the line" begins.

Some people will allow touching above the waist, others allow touching below the waist. Some will even allow oral sex, because *it's not sex, right? Even though it has the word* sex *in it.*

Some come up with a viable solution, rubbing against each other with clothes on. The term I always heard was *dry humping.* I think couples feel a little less guilty with this one because there is no actual touching of hands to skin . . . although couples who engage in this activity can actually bring each other to climax.

This is getting a little explicit and uncomfortable for some of us reading, but these are the lines that young people search for. And most of them figure it out on their own . . . *because very few Christians talk about it explicitly.*

So most will continue to wonder, *How far is too far?*

Loopholes

When I was in high school, I was one of the believers in "no sex until marriage." But everything else was fair game.

Oh, I didn't truly believe that. In all honesty, in the back of my mind I figured that oral sex was probably wrong, and I didn't even allow myself to consider the morality of any "below the waist" activity.

So during those years I made sexual decisions using blurred lines and messy morality. I "kind of" knew some of it was wrong, but I definitely didn't know where the line was.

Whenever we talked about sex in youth group, I was curious. In hindsight, I think I was looking for a stamp of approval more than anything else. Like a Pharisee, I wanted to see a list of do's and don'ts . . . *and look for a loophole.* I had a talent for finding loopholes. (I should have been a lawyer.)

I remember hearing sex talks where they told me that "petting" was bad. I can barely type that word without shuddering. Man, that word is awkward. But for some reason youth workers in the eighties used it. "Don't do it," they told us. But I never heard a good explanation for why, other than the fact that the girl's dad would find out and hunt me down (which is a pretty compelling reason, I might add).

So I remember walking away from these discussions thinking, *Okay, no hands touching below the waist.*

But "dry humping" was fair game!

A loophole!

No one ever taught me the explicit truth. And yes, the Bible is very explicit on the subject.

So please allow me to say something again, something I've been repeating all through the book. We need to talk about this explicitly with our kids. Our kids are hearing explicit lies, and we're the ones who can tell them the explicit truth.

So how can we help our kids answer the question, "*How far can I go?*"

Try talking about baseball.

Sex Is a Process

Sex isn't just intercourse. It starts way before that. Consider the proverbial baseball analogy.

"I got to third base with her."

If you can reflect back to a time when you were in a middle school boys' locker room or sat at a table in the school cafeteria surrounded by your friends, you've probably heard about *the bases.*

Of course there is no reference book. *The bases* were just explained to us on the playground some day when we were young.

First base is kissing.

Second base is touching above the waist.

Third base is touching below the waist, and maybe includes oral sex in most circles.

A home run is "going all the way" or "intercourse," to use the scientific term.

Maybe we didn't hear about the bases all at once, but we've heard them referred to.

The analogy is actually pretty good, because in baseball you round the bases; you don't just run straight to third. A guy usually doesn't walk up to his girlfriend and just stick his hands down her pants. If so, he'll be slapped and called a pig.

We have an official term for rounding the bases: *foreplay.*

As you know, sex isn't just intercourse. Sex is a process that starts with passionate kissing, progresses to embracing, touching . . . and eventually ends with intercourse.

Lovers never start with intercourse. It's impossible, really. The body doesn't work like that. A rapist goes straight to intercourse, and not only hurts a woman emotionally because of the lack of consent, but most often does all kinds of damage physically because her body wasn't ready for it.

So why all these graphic details?

Because it's important for our teens to understand sexuality and how the body works. Sex is a beautiful process that begins with foreplay and peaks at intercourse. Help your kids understand this process. (I go through these same examples in my book to teens, *Sex Matters*.)

Why Is It So Difficult to Stop?

Anyone who has been alone with someone they are attracted to and allowed the process to start knows that it is like trying to stop a raging fire!

So why is it so difficult to stop?

Because it's not supposed to be stopped!

The truth is, God made this process so that when a husband sees his wife wearing something sexy, his motor starts running.

They kiss and embrace. Soon, his pulse will accelerate, his penis will grow erect (keeping it in scientific terms), and her vagina will start to lubricate naturally. They might touch each other intimately, caressing various parts of the body, places no other person touches, places reserved for a husband and a wife. Eventually the man will insert his penis into her vagina, and the two will eagerly move in a motion that provides stimulation to both male and female until one or both climax.

The whole process is amazing and euphoric . . . and yes, a little awkward to talk about. After all, it is an intimate act designed for a husband and wife to share privately.

So why the human anatomy and sexuality lesson?

We need to help our kids understand that this process is for marriage. The entire process is only for marriage.

I can hear it now. *"What? Are you saying kissing is only for marriage?"*

I've heard that question. I've heard it from the boy who was just like me, the boy who wants to know the exact line so he can find a loophole. Some kids might as well ask us to provide them a list of what you can and can't do.

The Legalist's List

Kissing—*yes*

Hugging—*yes*

Hand to fully clothed breasts—*no*

Hand to genitals—*no*

Big toe to kneecap—*as long as you are wearing socks*

Jumping rope—*sounds fun, so no*

This is ridiculous. Whenever we start making up lists of rules, we tend to look less like Jesus and more like the Pharisees. The Pharisees made huge lists and were still corrupt. Don't provide your kids with a list. Do them one better. Teach them how to understand truth and make wise decisions based on good information.

The truth is, God wants us to share the intimate process of sex within marriage. We learned that in the last chapter. No one who has even a remedial understanding of Scripture would argue that. The argument always arises with *"How far can I go?"*

Don't Start the Process

I just proposed that unmarried couples shouldn't even begin the process.

"Prove it!" I would have declared when I was a teenager.

Okay. Exhibit A: *Jesus' teaching on lust.*

Remember this passage from the last chapter? Jesus himself addressed lust, labeling it just as sinful as adultery.

> You have heard the commandment that says, "You must not commit adultery." But I say, anyone who even looks at a woman with lust has already committed adultery with her in his heart.
>
> Matthew 5:27–28

Do you know any young man who can lie on top of his girlfriend, passionately kiss her and grope her breasts (second base) . . . and not lust?

Seriously. What is going through this guy's mind at the moment? Is he thinking about feeding homeless people? Is he thinking about his math homework? Not a chance.

His mind is 110 percent focused on her body and how much he wants it. Everything within him wants to go further.

It's hard to deny this kind of excitement, because the body will evidence the excitement in so many ways. God designed it perfectly so. When a couple gets into an intimate situation, heartbeats quicken, adrenaline flows through the bloodstream, the penis hardens, and the vagina gets wet. The human bodies start preparing for one of the greatest physical pleasures imaginable, an intimate bond that a husband and wife can share uniquely together. Dopamine rushes through the brain, stimulating even greater pleasure, and oxytocin is secreted by the posterior pituitary gland, inspiring greater bonding.

The bodies get excited and begin this sexually intimate process that prepares them for intercourse. This whole process is a good thing when you are married. At the same time, this is something we shouldn't *initiate* before we're married.

I think of the classic show *Everybody Loves Raymond*. In one episode, Raymond was walking around in his boxers while cleaning the house, and his wife, Debra, walked into the room, noticed him cleaning, and got turned on. (Yes, that is the key to a woman's heart. Get off your butt and do something around the house!) She walked up to him, whispered in his ear, and began kissing him passionately.

Suddenly, she heard a sound upstairs from the kids and stopped her sexual advance. Frustrated with Debra, Raymond exclaimed, "What are you doing?! You can't stop. You already initiated the launch sequence!"

That's the best advice we can give our kids.

Don't even initiate the launch sequence.

No, I'm *not* telling our kids *they can't kiss*. In fact, I often word it the same way I worded it in my advice to guys in my book *The Guy's Guide to God, Girls, and the Phone in Your Pocket:* "Don't do anything with your girlfriend you wouldn't do in front of your grandmother."

It's like this: You're a teenage guy and your family throws a big dinner for your birthday, inviting the entire extended family and your girlfriend. After dinner you open presents. Your girlfriend gives you a really nice gift and you lean over and give her a kiss in front of everyone. She blushes, the adults smile, and your little brother exclaims, "Ew, gross!"

Sounds innocent.

Now picture the exact same scenario, same crowd, same present from the girlfriend . . . but this time, when you lean over and kiss her, you start becoming a little more passionate. Instead of just kissing her, you crawl on top of her and start kissing her neck and breathing heavy.

Who would do this?

Chances are Dad might spray you with the garden hose!

Why wouldn't a teenage guy do this in front of Grandma and the whole family?

Perhaps because it's . . . *intimate.* And intimate situations like this usually progress to something else. The world teaches us, *Who cares if it progresses to something else?* But God's design is that intimate situations like this are really reserved for two people who have committed to each other for life in marriage.

The Wrong Question

I commonly hear young people ask, "How far is too far?" That's like asking me, "How close to the fire can I get without getting burned?" Sadly, the only way to find out is to *get burned.*

News flash: We don't have to learn everything in life the hard way.

So whenever a young couple asks me, "How far should we go?" I respond, "You're asking me the wrong question."

The better question is, "How far can we stay away?"

Let's look at the situation. From what we've discussed so far, most of us have concluded a few things:

1. God's design is the best way; therefore, our kids should *want to wait* until marriage for sex.
2. Sex isn't just intercourse—it's the whole process. After all, Jesus said lusting is the same as actually doing it.
3. No one should initiate the process unless they're married—because the process is meant to be finished. And there's only one person our kids should start and finish the process with—their spouse!

With these things in mind, encourage your kids to ask, "How can I be successful in saving myself for my spouse?"

Sex is a huge temptation for young people today, and not just couples, but anyone:

- the twelve-year-old gamer sitting in front of the computer;
- the twenty-one-year-old college student invited to go clubbing with her friends;
- the sixteen-year-old high school fullback who is being encouraged by all his buddies to "get laid";

- the fifteen-year-old girlfriend who is feeling pressure from her boyfriend.

The world is screaming "Just do it!" And our kids' bodies aren't always disagreeing.

The biggest issue many young people are going to have to address is, *Do I want to live for the truth and make godly choices, or live for the quick thrill of the moment?*

Those who want to stay pure need to realize the draw of sexual temptation and avoid it at all costs.

Maybe that's why the Bible often uses the word *flee*.

Fleeing

Sometimes I use the following illustration when talking about fleeing.

Fact: Dentists have recommended that a toothbrush be kept at least six feet away from a toilet to avoid airborne particles resulting from the flush.

How many of you are going to store your toothbrush just five feet away? It's only a foot shorter than the dentist recommends. Maybe only a few urine particles will splash onto your toothbrush.

How many of you are going to store it right next to the toilet by the toilet paper roll? You could build a little shelf right there.

How many of you want to hang it by a string in the toilet bowl so that it is practically rinsed every time you flush?

The thing about the subject of sexual temptation that always amuses me is the amount of risk people are willing to take. Actually, using the word *risk* isn't accurate. The thing about this subject that always amuses me is how *stupid* we are willing to be just to fulfill an urge.

Sadly, people often leave their brains at home when they embark on sexual decisions. It's foolish to wait until we're in a sexual situation to decide what we're going to do. Almost any person is going to choose sex when *in the situation*. It's the way God wired us.

So maybe we should listen to the Bible's advice and "flee" sexual immorality and lustful pleasures.

If we're told that we shouldn't put our toothbrush within six feet of the toilet because of airborne particles . . . most of us will probably store our toothbrush about twenty feet away if possible. Why? Because the thought of poop fumes or pee splashes wandering onto our toothbrushes is *not acceptable*!

There is a principle here: If we discover danger to be within a certain proximity, we avoid that proximity completely.

Why don't we do that with sexual temptation? We determine we don't even want to start the process . . . then we go and put ourselves in situations where the process not only starts, but it's hard to stop!

Why flirt with disaster?

Help your kids understand God's design. They need to be careful not to initiate launch sequence. Encourage them to save the amazing process of sex for marriage, and "flee" sexual temptation.

We'll talk a little more about what fleeing actually looks like day-to-day in chapter 8, but first let's look at some specifics about each gender.

Your Daughter

More than just a sex object

Have you shopped for Halloween costumes for your daughter recently?

My own teenage girls love costumes, so they are quick to grab the Party City costume insert in the paper each week during the month of October. The front page always features some of the popular costumes for girls. Naughty Nurse. Racy Referee. I'm not making this up. Some of these might as well be in the Victoria's Secret catalog.

Whatever happened to good ol' princess costumes? *Anyone?* How about a clown?

Halloween is one of those times where the pressure is on young girls to be sexy. Cady nailed it in the cult classic film *Mean Girls* when she said, "In the regular world, Halloween is when children dress up in costumes and beg for candy. In Girl World, Halloween is the one night a year when a girl can dress like a total slut and no other girls can say anything about it."

If you don't believe me, just Google "teenage Halloween costumes" and click on the first thing you see. Rows upon rows of the same slinky outfits.

These are for teenagers?

And who says our girls are going to just shop in the "teen section" of the catalog? Most high school girls won't hesitate to flip the page, browsing through the costumes for all ages. How about Mile High Captain or Dirty Cop? (I don't have to explain what these costumes look like, do I?)

Can we please stop marketing this stuff to our kids?

Now, I don't want to be a whiner or a complainer—there are enough of them around. But at what point do moms and dads need to just step in and say "No"?

Seriously . . . when?

Too Sexy Too Soon

Sadly, this problem is not unique to Halloween. If you've been to a mall or flipped through the clothing ads lately, you've noticed that most girls' clothing has become increasingly skimpier and sexier, prompting many parents to question, *Is this making our daughters too sexy too soon?*

We could point fingers at the extreme examples like Abercrombie & Fitch, who not only have been criticized for selling thong underwear in children's sizes with the words "eye candy" and "wink wink," but also came under fire when they marketed push-up triangle bikini tops to girls as young as seven. (What exactly would second-grade girls push up?) Sure, Abercrombie is guilty of being ultra-risqué . . . but have you shopped for girls' clothing at *any* store lately?

I go shopping with my daughters often, and let me just say . . . *It's becoming more and more difficult to find modest clothes.* Some parents are getting fed up with this corporate pedophilia.

Don't worry, I'm not one of those dads who is making his daughter wear turtlenecks and full-length skirts that cover the ankles, but at the same time, I'm not really excited about how *short* shorts are actually getting. And how provocative do tops have to be? Today's dads find themselves asking, *Am I comfortable with my daughter's cleavage hanging out?*

The fashion world is putting the pressure on, nudging young girls to get too sexy too soon, and most girls have opted in.

Scratch that.

Most *parents* have opted in. It would be a little narrow of me to put the blame on our kids, or on clothing companies that pimp this kind of stuff to our daughters, when it is we, the parents of these girls, who are "lowering the bar" and actually purchasing it. This is yet another instance when parents need to consider the consequences that go along with lowering their standards like this.

Perhaps we need to stop lowering the bar.

Sexualization

We're witnessing the symptoms of a society that values sexuality over other characteristics. It's what the American Psychological Association (APA) defines as "sexualization."

It starts with the normal feelings of insecurity.

Am I pretty enough?

Do I measure up?

These are the questions young girls ask themselves when they look in the mirror, touching up makeup, running the flatiron through their hair that one last time, trying to make it perfect. Any father of teen and tween girls has witnessed this. Even the most beautiful of today's young girls often struggle with feelings of "too fat," "too much acne," "small boobs," etc.

Where are they getting these ideas? What kind of standard are they trying to measure up to?

Psychologist and author Vivian Diller, PhD, gives us some insight in her article "Sex and the Single Teen: Internet Porn and Body Image":

> I believe the distorted, enhanced imagery burdens teenage girls with unrealistic expectations about beauty and body image and with damaging ideas about what is attractive and sexually appealing to

> others. From the perfect waif-like models in teen magazines to the perfectly voluptuous ones on internet porn, the common theme is that these body shapes are unrealistic and unattainable.[1]

So what do our girls do when they feel like they can't measure up? Enter "sexualization" stage left.

The APA actually released a report titled, "The Sexualization of Girls," defining sexualization as "When a person's value comes only from his or her sexual appeal or behavior, to the exclusion of other characteristics . . . a person is sexually objectified—that is, made into a thing for another's sexual use."[2]

If you want to see examples of this, just click on any of the most popular music videos on iTunes or YouTube (our kids are). You'll see plenty of women dressed in hyper-sexualized outfits.

Why? Is their dancing alone not good enough? Are the vocals not compelling enough? Do we need to sprinkle in a little bit of sexually provocative material to spice it up?

Lady Gaga readily admits to using these kinds of tactics: "I was 19 and I was playing a show where I was supposed to debut all this new material. When I sat down to play I couldn't get everyone to stop talking so I took off all my clothes. Works every time."[3]

Anyone who has seen Lady Gaga perform has witnessed this sexualization. She is an amazing singer and entertainer, but, to borrow from the APA's definition, she continues to "value her sexual appeal and behavior" over other characteristics. Gaga is sexually objectified in most of her music videos.

Our daughters are bombarded with these subtle media messages daily, clearly communicating: *You need to be sexy. You need to dress risqué.* If they walk through the mall, the posters are screaming the same messages: *You need to be thin. You need to have perfect skin. You need to show cleavage.*

Our daughters are slowly becoming sexualized.

According to the APA's research, the consequences of sexualization are "negative effects in a variety of domains, including cognitive functioning, physical and mental health, sexuality and attitudes and beliefs."

As parents, we've probably seen these effects firsthand. Many of our daughters are buying the lies of the media. The media is offering sexualization as the solution to insecurity.

It works like this, girls think: *Guys notice me when I'm overtly sexual* (revealing tops, short shorts, provocative words and actions), *and being noticed is what I want, right?*

The world is beginning to value sexual appeal and behavior to the exclusion of other characteristics. It's up to parents to teach their daughters what is truly valuable.

Teaching Our Girls They Are Valuable

How do we teach our daughters that they are not sex objects? I mean, seriously. What does this actually look like?

I see four ways to teach our girls that their value isn't determined by their sex appeal.

1. Teach Our Daughters to Recognize Lies

Our daughters are bombarded with lies far more than they hear the truth. We need to teach them to recognize these clever lies.

Think about the typical day for the average teenage girl and how much of her time involves listening to music. The average eight- to eighteen-year-old in America listens to two hours and thirty-one minutes of music per day.[4] Do you want to know what they're listening to? Look at your daughter's favorite playlist on her phone. If she's like most of the girls today, that list might look a lot like the top music on Spotify, iTunes, or the Billboard Hot 100 at any given time. I'm looking at that list right now, and it's full of songs with two basic themes:

- the desire for temporary pleasures (sex, money, fame, status, etc.)
- pain and regret

Interestingly enough, the first category is usually full of lies, telling listeners that the quick thrill is worth it, and consequences are rarely seen. The second category, however, often tells the truth, expressing the feelings of pain, loneliness, and regret (often the result of the activities in the first category).

Let's take a look at a prominent song from each category. Katy Perry's "Last Friday Night" is a perfect example of a song from the last decade that focuses on the temporary thrills in life. Why is this song a big deal? Well, Perry's 2010 album *Teenage Dream* made history in 2011 when "Last Friday Night" went number one, the fifth song on the album to do so. No artist has done that since Michael Jackson in the eighties. Perry was the first female artist to achieve that.

Like much of Katy's work, the song and video were really well done, but they were also chock-full of subtle lies that young people consumed a gallon at a time.

The lyrics say it all, opening with the line, "There's a stranger in my bed."

Unfortunately, the song only digresses, talking about streaking, skinny dipping, and having a ménage à trois. Since the song didn't have any actual swear words, it wasn't labeled "EXPLICIT" and it played in every WalMart, Target, and school campus that played music.

As the song ends, Katy says she'll do it all again "next Friday night."

This is a great illustration of the irresponsible lyrics that our teenagers marinate in daily. The message is clear: Enjoy all these risky behaviors (sleep with a stranger, streak, skinny dip, do a threesome, break the law), and after reflecting on your experience, *plan on doing it all over again*.

The subtle message is, "These temporary thrills are worth it." (I don't know how accurate it is to even call these messages "subtle." They are pretty obvious.)

That's just one of the most popular songs from the last decade. You'll find plenty just like it (or much worse) in the top playlists young people stream today.

But there's a second category of music that our girls are hearing, and that's the music that expresses pain and regret. Adele's award-winning album *21* is a sample of this category. This well-written album reveals the real pain that Adele felt during a breakup. Listeners related to feelings of loneliness, hurt, and regret. That's probably why it was the best-selling album in 2011 and 2012, won a Grammy for "Album of the Year" in 2012, and in 2014 became the first-ever digital album to sell three million copies.

Songs like these always frequent the charts. Consider Eminem and Rihanna's song and music video "Love the Way You Lie," a graphic depiction of the pain and abuse that some endure in relationships. Or look at Pink's "Perfect." This music video paints a realistic picture of a girl who never felt like she measured up to the expectations put on her. (My older daughter, Alyssa, and I actually had a great talk after watching that video together.)

The pain and hurt expressed in most of these songs is very authentic. The problem is, most of these songs don't provide any answers, just questions, and many times a nostalgic look back on temporary thrills that helped the artist endure the pain.

You can learn a lot from the music your kids stream from their phones. I often have told parents at my parenting workshops, "The iPhone is the window to the heart." That's why it's good for parents to always have the passwords to their kids' phones. A quick glimpse at the most played songs in their music library can tell you a lot.

It's important to have frequent discussions with our daughters about what they're listening to and teach them how to make good entertainment media decisions. These conversations will be stifled if we "freak out." So remember what we discussed in chapter 3 about creating a climate that cultivates conversations. We need to raise their awareness about the lies they are being exposed to, and equip them to recognize lies and search for the truth.

I think of the passage of Scripture where Paul is encouraging the people of Ephesus to be unified and grow in maturity in Christ. He tells them, when they mature in their knowledge in Christ . . .

> Then we will no longer be immature like children. We won't be tossed and blown about by every wind of new teaching. We will not be influenced when people try to trick us with lies so clever they sound like the truth.
>
> Ephesians 4:14

Parents need to guide their daughters on this road to maturity, helping them recognize the lies that sound like the truth. I've talked with my daughters about sexualization. I point it out when I see it. More important, I ask them questions to get them to start recognizing lies and thinking through the consequences.

Moms and dads can do this while walking through the mall together:

"What do you think the dress on that mannequin is communicating to guys?"

"Do you think girls really want to communicate that?"

"What are some of the consequences that could result from communicating that message?"

You can ask questions while watching TV or movies together:

"Why do you think he is trying so hard to get her to come back to his apartment?"

"We know that sex is an awesome gift God has given to married couples; what are some of the consequences of having sex with just anyone you meet at a bar?"

"Do you think she was looking for sex or for love?"

The key is to frequently engage our kids in meaningful conversations. Make these conversations a *dialogue*, not a *monologue*. Use plenty of thought-provoking questions that get them talking and us listening (my previous book, *Get Your Teenagers Talking*, provides you with 180 of these discussion springboards).

This doesn't mean we should point out girls in short skirts and say, "Look at those sluts!" Far from it. Walk that line Jesus walked: compassionate toward the lost, yet not afraid to stand for the truth. So be careful not to be judgmental or condescending toward others when you're helping your own kids understand modesty.

Ask girls questions so that they'll begin to recognize lies when they see them. Your goal is to prepare them for the day they leave your house and are making these decisions on their own. Are you preparing them for that day? Does your daughter spot sexualization when she sees it?

There is a second way to teach our girls that their value stretches way beyond sex appeal.

2. Help Our Girls Recognize True Value

In the same way we help them recognize lies, we need to help them recognize the truth.

In a world full of lies, parents need to become a source of truth. The world tells our daughters that outward appearance and sexiness are of the utmost importance, but parents can and should teach their daughters that their value comes from much more than sex appeal and sexual behavior. In fact, "People judge by outward appearance, but the Lord looks at the heart" (1 Samuel 16:7).

If we go back to the APA's definition of sexualization, we'll notice that the world tends to value our daughters' "sexual appeal or behavior, to the exclusion of other characteristics." We can help our daughters begin to know and experience that they are so much more than sex objects by encouraging them in those "other characteristics."

Does she like singing? Give her voice lessons.

Does she show artistic promise? Let her try some art classes.

Is she an athlete? Sign her up for soccer. Give her the chance to experience the camaraderie of being on a team.

Did she get good grades? Take her out for a family celebration when her report card comes out.

Help your daughter understand that life is much more than just being a sex object. Affirm her in her values, skills, and behaviors.

Yes . . . I just used the word *values*.

Sports, school, and art can be really rewarding activities, but don't forget to affirm your daughter where it matters most . . . her character. Who she is inside.

Teach your daughter to live for eternity, not temporary pleasures. The world loves to focus on the now, pretending there are no consequences. Sadly, the consequences always do come.

We need to teach our daughters the joy of living a life of faith, one that recognizes there is much more to this world than just the temporary stuff we see all around us.

Hebrews 11:1 defines faith in a way that looks beyond the quick thrill: "Faith is the confidence that what we hope for will actually happen; it gives us assurance about things we cannot see."

Sometimes we get distracted by temporary pleasures. Other times we grow fatigued with struggles. That's where faith comes in. We can teach our daughters that the drama, struggles, and trials they're experiencing are only temporary and are shaping them to be women of God! We can help them learn to live with an eternal focus.

When our daughters start living for God instead of for themselves, they'll experience an incredible joy.

Affirm your daughter when she shares, talks respectfully, or obeys. Catch her doing something right. All the while, be looking for her areas of strength. If you see she is gifted in the area of compassion, give her an opportunity to use it and experience the joy God gives when we serve him in our strengths.

Mission trips and service opportunities are great ways to help our daughters see true value. Every time our family has helped serve food to homeless people through our church, I've noticed something. Not only do my kids get a chance to make a difference in someone else's life, but they forget about their own trivial problems and insecurities for an evening as they selflessly serve others.

Funny how that works. When God uses us to reach out to the poor and needy, our own issues just don't seem like such a big deal.

Encourage your daughter to look for these values in a future spouse as well. The world is constantly telling us that men should be rich, powerful, athletic, or the life of the party. As your daughter matures, ask her what qualities she would like to see in her future spouse. Ask her if she had the choice of athleticism or commitment to marriage, which would she choose? Help her look for values like compassion, spiritual maturity, integrity, and a passion for God. Help her look for a guy who wants more than just sex.

Look for every opportunity to help your daughter begin to know and experience that she is much more than a sex object.

3. Teach Girls to Dress Modestly

Another way to do this is to teach modesty and discretion.

Earlier in this chapter I pointed the finger back at ourselves. It's parents who have lowered the bar and allowed their daughters to buy in to the lie of sexualization. And it's up to parents to step in and say, "No, you don't need to wear that low-cut top and show your cleavage to get the attention of guys. That's the wrong kind of attention."

This isn't easy. It's hard to find clothes that aren't overtly sexual, and at the same time . . . aren't hideously ugly.

How can we teach our girls to walk this line?

We could be like the one mother we all know at church who always dresses her daughter in Amish-like apparel. I know her daughter well. (I've met hundreds of them when I was speaking at camps and youth events across the country.) When this young girl turns eighteen, she's most likely going to rebel completely. She's already started.

Or I guess we can do the opposite and be like the overly permissive parents of many of the girls we see on public high school campuses—girls who hardly wear anything at all.

Parents have a choice to make. Are we supposed to sway to either of these extremes? Is there a modest balance?

First, I don't think we need to overreact to either extreme mentioned above. Personally, I don't see the need to wrap up our girls head to toe. I've had numerous conversations with my girls about the way they dress, explaining to them the simple truth that it affects the guys around them. I've talked about how visual guys are and how short skirts and revealing tops really affect them. Dads can offer a unique perspective to their daughters. They can give their girls a glimpse into the mind of a guy.

This isn't just one conversation. Parents should regularly engage in these conversations when they read an article or see an example in the media. Don't lecture in these situations; instead, ask questions. When I first read the APA's sexualization report, I used it as an opportunity for dialogue, asking my girls their opinion on the subject. I asked them questions like:

"What are some examples you see of sexualization?"

"Why do you think girls buy in to this lie that they are only valuable as sex objects?"

"How can girls avoid selling out to this lie?"

"What are some specific actions you might need to take this week to avoid selling out to this lie?"

The goal is to teach our kids good decision making so they can eventually make these choices on their own, hopefully with plenty of opportunities to try out some of this decision making while still in the home. In our house, these have been good conversations.

Does that mean we never had disagreements about apparel in my house? Ha! I wish. We had to remind our girls quite often, helping them choose modest clothing.

My girls didn't always agree with our rules, but that's okay. We set realistic guidelines, discussed them together, and explained why they existed. Most of the time, my girls were pretty cool with that.

When they were younger, we bought their clothes for them, teaching them modesty and engaging in frequent conversations about it. As they became older, we let them make many of these decisions on their own so they could experience the decision-making process.

Every once in a great while we stepped in with veto power, but rarely. Once our daughters were seventeen and a half, they made all these decisions completely on their own.

We called it "no rules at seventeen and a half." The concept is simple. We started strict when our girls were little, but we slowly lightened up with our guidelines, teaching them to make decisions on their own. At seventeen and a half, while they still lived at home, they experienced "no rules."

Yes, some people thought we were crazy. But think about it. When kids are eighteen years old they can join the Marines, move out, and do whatever they want! Why not prepare them for that power just six months early while they are still living in the safety of our home? We can't make all the decisions for our kids their entire lives. We need to prepare them to make good decisions on their own.

Are you teaching your girls how to dress modestly?

Will they choose to dress modestly when they are in their college dorm choosing their own outfits?

Remember the big picture. We're trying to teach our daughters they have *waaaaaaaay* more value than just their sexuality.

There is one more way I've found to teach our girls that they are valuable.

4. Teach Our Daughters They Are Beautiful

"Show me a girl who dresses like that, and I'll show you a girl whose father was absent." That's what my friend Ray said. I didn't believe him when he said it. I thought the statement was dogmatic and shallow. *How can he make such a generalization!*

I was only a few years into youth ministry and hadn't spent much time with teenagers. Years passed, and as my wife and I ministered to a growing number of teenage girls who dressed risqué and craved sexual attention, we began to notice a common denominator: *the absent dad.*

Perhaps Ray was right.

The most common example was the dad who was literally absent. He either abandoned the family or never saw the kids because of the way the divorce or separation was finalized. Mom was left to raise the kids, and in many cases, the young girl began seeking male attention wherever she could get it.

This is sad to witness. Girls want to be noticed. Dads who are absent leave a void.

But sometimes we saw the phenomena of the *emotionally absent* dad. Dad was in the living room but he never talked to his daughter, never went to her softball games, and never told her she was beautiful. These dads weren't much better than the *physically absent* dads. Their daughters were just as desperate for attention, and if Dad wasn't giving it, they sought it elsewhere.

Don't get me wrong; I'm not discounting the power of Mom here. Mom's role is huge and vitally important. In fact, she typically will be the one having more of those conversations mentioned above about modesty as they shop together and have girl-to-girl time. And moms can definitely help affirm their girls' beauty as well. But I'm going to focus more attention on dads in this fourth way we can teach our girls value, because dads have the unique role of demonstrating to our girls how they should be treated by men.

Dads, one way we can do this is by "dating" our daughters.

Don't let the word *date* scare you. Dads have the opportunity to take their daughters out for lunch, movies, mini golf, hiking . . . you name it. Show your girls how they are supposed to be treated by a male.

I'm far from a perfect dad, but once, Ashley, my youngest, was telling her sister about a guy who didn't open the door for her "like Dad does." She saw me opening the car door for my wife when our family went out for dinner and she thought, *I'm going to find me a man like that.*

That made me feel pretty good.

When we date our daughters, listen to them, laugh with them, and pay attention to them . . . *we respect them for who they truly are*. Our attention to them affirms them in the areas of their true beauty. And that makes our girls feel pretty special.

Dads can make a huge difference in the lives of their kids.

Sometimes dads make the mistake of taking the backseat in raising their kids. We can't. Girls need their daddies. All too often, Daddy isn't there, physically or emotionally. I witnessed this sad situation too many times to count in my twenty years of youth ministry. And I still see it today in the lives of many of my own daughters' friends. It's a little scary how physical some of these young girls get and how comfortable they are with *any* male attention.

I heard someone say, "If dads don't touch their daughters, other guys will."

I remember thinking that sounded a little creepy. I don't like thinking about a father's compassionate, loving touch in comparison to the hormone-induced touch of some pubescent boyfriend.

But realistically, if dads don't hug their daughters, demonstrating true love and affection . . . their daughters will look for it in the wrong places.

I think many fathers underestimate the impact they have on their kids.

U.S. News highlighted a review of thirteen different studies about the effect fathers had on the sexual behavior of their kids. The review found the father's role significant in kids' development. In fact, all thirteen studies suggested that "communication between fathers and kids is especially influential."[5]

As I was writing this, I took my friend Travis to lunch and asked him how to counter this tendency for girls to act out sexually. Travis is a psychologist and has counseled families for years. Without any hesitation he responded, "Dad having a good relationship with his daughter so she has value for who she is. Today's girls need males who model healthy relationships."

I pushed back a little bit. "What about single moms?"

"Get your daughter involved in youth group, sports, etc., where they can encounter good male role models. Maybe an uncle, coach, teacher, etc."

Single moms need to be very selective about who they date and who they bring into the house as a role model. Is this a man you want influencing your kids?

In Dr. Meg Meeker's book *Strong Fathers, Strong Daughters*, she contends that a daughter's relationship with her dad is much more important than most people realize. "To become a strong, confident woman, a daughter needs her father's attention, protection, courage, and wisdom."

It's as simple as this: *Our girls need to hear that they are beautiful*. They need to feel safe. They need male attention and advice. They can either hear it from their dads . . . *or they'll seek it somewhere else*.

Dads need to do more than just tell their daughters that they are beautiful; they need to *treat them* like they're beautiful. This is much deeper than just opening the car door for them (although that's a great practice). This means devoting ourselves to something that most men are terrible at: *noticing*.

Men need to learn the secret of noticing. This simple but amazing tool opens up doors in any relationship (marriage, friendships), but it works especially well with teenage girls because:

1. They crave to be noticed . . .

and . . .

2. Not a lot of people take time to notice them . . . *other than predators.*

Scary thought, huh?

Okay, I'll step off my soapbox about dads. Moms can help build value in this area as well. After all, noticing is a powerful tool. Both moms and dads can say "I love you" and "You are beautiful" in a more powerful way by simply noticing. Here are some examples of noticing your daughter throughout the day:

NOTICE HER HAIR OR MAKEUP IN A POSITIVE WAY.

What to do: "Wow, I like that color eyeliner; it really brings out your gorgeous eyes!"

What not to do: "Did you do something different with your hair?" (Moms would probably vouch for me here that we should never ask a question to a female that is subject to interpretation. Especially a pubescent female!)

SIT DOWN WITH HER AND JUST LISTEN

What to do: If your daughter is sitting at the kitchen table eating a snack by herself, sit down with her, look her in the eyes, and ask her, "So what's been the best part of your day so far?" If that works, you can follow up with "What's been the worst?"

What not to do: Don't ask a question as you pass by. Instead, sit down and look her in the eyes, giving her your full attention.

NOTICE HER OUTFIT

What to do: "That jacket is really cute on you. Is that new? Wow, I like it."

What not to do: "What made you wear that?" (Again, I've learned to never ask a question to a female that hints skepticism. The best way to play it safe is to realize that your daughter might be on the edge of tears about her outfit and could cry at any moment!)

Show up at her sporting events or plays

What to do: Show up, cheer, and take her out for a fun snack afterward.

What not to do: Don't make the mistake of believing her when she tells you, "You don't have to come." Be there anyway. She might not even realize that she wants you there.

Buy her something that you know she wants

What to do: If you see her consistently looking at a pair of shoes in a catalog or the Sunday ads, then surprise her and buy her the shoes. Or better yet, say, "I noticed you've been eyeing those Vans in the Sunday ads. Whadaya say we go out and get them, and then get some ice cream on the way home!"

What not to do: Don't just guess at what she wants. Only buy something if you know she wants it. Or you can take her shopping and let her choose. Take notice of what she likes for next time.

When we take the time to notice our girls, we are telling them we love them and care about them. We are telling them that they are valuable!

—

More Valuable Than . . .

A dad walked up to me after one of my parent workshops and we began dialoguing about how important it is to show our daughters they are valuable. He shared with me a story that happened in his home.

He described his relationship with his daughter as "so-so." The two of them talked occasionally, but never really deep. This dad didn't point the blame at anyone but himself. "I wasn't always the best listener," he shared candidly. "But then something happened last summer.

"My daughter came to me when I was working on the family's bills," he explained. "My kids had learned not to bug me during this time, sort of an unspoken rule. But for some reason, my daughter needed to talk, saw me sitting there with my checkbook open, with my bank statements and calculator all spread across the kitchen table. She simply said, 'Dad, I need to talk.'

"And that's when it happened," he said with a nod. "I don't know why I did this simple little gesture, but for some reason, I took my hand and slid all my paperwork aside, placed my elbows on the table, and said, 'Sure, sit down.'

"She sat down, we had the most amazing talk, and then I finished doing the bills. The conversation probably only took about twenty minutes, but it changed our relationship."

"How?" I asked curiously.

"She told her mom about it later that night. She said, 'Dad actually moved the bills aside and just listened.' There was something about me physically sliding all that stuff aside that communicated to her, *You are more important than all this stuff!* It changed our relationship forever. We can talk now like we've never talked before."

I'll never forget this guy's simple little experience.

Sometimes it's the simple gestures that tell our daughters, *You are valuable.*

What do you need to slide out of the way?

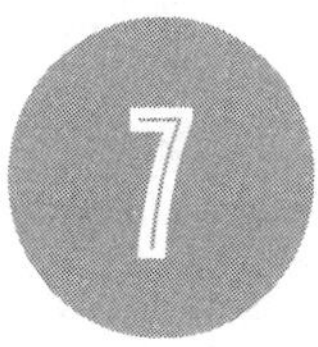

Your Son

More than just a sex drive

Raising a boy can be a fun experience for a parent . . . and a frightening experience, especially when he looks to you for social cues on behavior.

No pressure, right?

But that's what young boys do. They look to adults for guidance on how to talk and behave.

Who is your son looking to?

I have a fun memory with my son, Alec, when he was nine years old. He had been asking to watch the movie *Godzilla* for years. I kept replying, "It's too scary. Maybe when you're older."

One day, after literally years of asking me, he begged me again, "Dad, am I old enough to watch *Godzilla* yet?"

I smiled and asked, "I don't know. Do you think you are?"

"Oh yes," he quickly responded. "I won't be scared one bit!"

That evening during dinner we revealed to the family that Alec and I were going to have a "man night" and watch a man's movie together. His younger sisters were a little disappointed, but I assured them they didn't want to be there, "because men like to lie around in their underwear on the couch when they watch movies."

My wife, Lori, teased me, "Yeah, a little too much! Try putting some pants on around the house, Jonathan!"

After dinner when it was time to start the movie, Alec came out of his room with a big smile on his face wearing just a pair of boxer briefs.

"Come on, Dad!" he announced. "Get in your underwear! It's time for *man night*!"

I'm not sure what I taught my son that night . . . but he taught me something. Even our most subtle cues are absorbed and imitated by our sons.

What are your kids learning from you?

My friend Julie decided to take an active role teaching her son Jeff how to treat a lady. She did this by going on dates with him. The two of them made it a regular habit to have "date night" together.

Julie was a lot of fun, but she also didn't hesitate to teach him manners. Jeff quickly learned to chew with his mouth closed and not talk when his mouth was full. Julie would wait for Jeff to open the car door and the restaurant door. Jeff became quite the polite young man.

Eventually, Julie let him plan the dates, giving him the opportunity to be the man. She said this was a lot of fun. Often, she didn't even know what was in store for the evening (although he usually ran it by Dad, since they were picking up the tab).

Our kids won't learn these habits and skills themselves. Parents teach these. And they can have a lot of fun in the process.

The Pseudo Parent

What happens if Dad doesn't have guys' night with his son? What if Mom doesn't date her son? Seriously, what would happen if Mom or Dad forfeited their calling as parents and decided life is too busy to spend time hanging out with their son? What if neither of them ever engage in casual conversations about life, friendship . . . even conversations about sex? If this happens, something else gladly slides into place and teaches young people all they need to know about these subjects. Something else raises our kids. A pseudo parent.

I'm referring to entertainment media and technology. If a dad doesn't teach his kids about sex, then Google will. If a mom doesn't have these conversations, then social media will gladly step up. Entertainment media and technology are readily available, and today's young people are soaking it in and marinating in it most waking hours.

Numbers can vary a little, but one of the most respected and quoted studies in the field (from the Kaiser Family Foundation) revealed the average eight- to eighteen-year-old devotes over 7.5 hours per day to entertainment media and technology.[1] That's a lot of TV, music, Internet, and video games. And each year, technology keeps advancing. Now most of these popular gadgets have Internet connections included. Smartphones, game systems, Blu-ray players, TVs . . . they all offer easy access to the web. It's no surprise to hear that a teenager used a smartphone to access the web, but what about these other popular devices? For example, a recent study showed that 61 percent of U.S. teens used their game systems to go online.[2]

In short . . . kids have a lot of distractions just a click away on almost every screen they frequent.

What do you think they are learning about sex from these sources?

What are our sons' favorite hip-hop artists teaching them about how to treat women?

Or if that isn't scary enough . . . what are our sons learning about women from some of the darker corners of the world wide web?

In chapter 9 we'll explore exactly how prevalent online porn is, and frankly . . . *it's frightening.* What's more frightening is the misinformation that porn spreads about human sexuality.

David Segal, in his *New York Times* article "Does Porn Hurt Children?" couldn't help but notice common cautionary advice from the academics he interviewed:

> "I have a son," says Professor Reid of U.C.L.A., "and I don't want him getting his information about human sexuality from Internet porn because the vast majority of such material contains fraudulent

> messages about sex—that all women have insatiable sexual appetites, for example."[3]

In the world of porn, every woman is a sex object, flawless, promiscuous, and unrestrained. Today's young men are beginning to think this is the norm.

In my work with teenagers, I've spent a lot of time with teenage guys on and off campus. In fact, my first decade of ministry was campus ministry, so many of these kids were *not* the kinds of kids you'd find at church on any given Sunday. I don't know whether to celebrate or mourn the fact that often these guys become quite free in how they talk around me, especially when they are in groups.

There have been countless times when these guys will have begun talking about a girl they met or know from school. At any second these conversations can digress to a sexual nature.

"Oh, she wants it. You can tell."

Sometimes I have to remind them, "Guys! Come on. I have daughters. You're talking about someone else's daughter!"

"Oh, sorry," they often say, sometimes adding, "But if you saw the way this girl dressed, you'd know what we were talking about. She definitely is advertising."

Sadly, I've seen the other side of this with my daughters' friends, many of them dressed just like they described. Most of these girls are *not* vixens sitting around thinking about sex. In fact, most are confused girls who really want to be accepted, and they've noticed provocative dress garners attention.

When Dad and Mom don't talk with their sons about this, sons will buy the readily available lies of the world.

So what can parents do to counter these media lies permeating the world our boys live in?

We need to teach our boys how to be men of God. I see three areas where we can specifically teach our boys to grow into men of God.

1. The Humility to Spot Lies

Boys without boundaries become increasingly vulnerable to the lies creeping around them every day.

The common response I hear from young men is, "Oh, don't worry. I don't pay attention to all that stuff," or "It doesn't affect me." So often they refuse to guard themselves.

It seems to me that males are more prone to deny these kinds of dangers, simply because boys tend to think they're bulletproof! Bulletproof sounds romantic when it's expressed as bravery, but scary when it becomes sheer carelessness. We've all met guys whose cavalier attitude is nothing more than an amalgamation of pride and foolishness.

Maybe that's why the Bible puts so much value on humility. Humility is a prerequisite for fleeing temptation. James says it well:

> But he gives us more grace. That is why Scripture says:
> "God opposes the proud
> but shows favor to the humble."
> Submit yourselves, then, to God. Resist the devil, and he will flee from you.
>
> James 4:6–7 NIV

A big part of recognizing the world's lies is recognizing our own vulnerability to those lies.

I've heard so many people quote verse 7 above . . . *but leave out the first part of the verse*. Someone will say, "As the Scriptures say, 'Resist the devil and he will flee from you.'"

No wonder so many people fail. The moment we see resisting temptation as a task we achieve on our own, we're destined for failure. Men especially can picture standing strong against great adversity like warriors fighting a great battle. It's a nice daydream . . . *but it's not what the Scripture says.*

The truth is, we need to get down on our knees and cry out to God, "I've tried to do this on my own so many times and failed miserably. I need your help. God, take over! You do this for me. Not my will, but yours."

We aren't bulletproof. We never have been. The great heroes of the Bible weren't bulletproof. Abraham pimped out his wife because he was scared for his own life. David committed adultery with the wife of one of his best men, then killed him to cover up his affair. And Solomon, the wisest man in the entire Bible, gave up on his faith because he disobeyed God directly and surrounded himself with women who worshiped other gods.

That's the way it usually happens. God warns us about a danger and we ignore his warnings.

Guys can learn a lot from looking at the life of Solomon. Solomon had all the potential in the world. By God's might, Israel was a powerful nation at the time, and God laid out some guidelines for his kings in Deuteronomy 17:14–20. He basically said . . .

If you're gonna have a king, choose an Israelite and make sure that he at least follows these simple guidelines:

1. Don't collect horses or chariots. If you do, nations might think that you're great because you have a bunch of horses and chariots. I want nations to know that you're great because of me, God!
2. Don't marry a bunch of wives. Kings often marry to create treaties with other nations. You don't need this, because you have me, God! Besides, these women will lure you to start worshiping their false gods instead of me.
3. Don't collect a bunch of silver or gold for yourself. You don't need gold to make you happy. I, God, give you all you need.
4. Have your king write a copy of the Scriptures for himself and read it every day. That way, he'll stay humble and won't turn from the truth.

That's all you need to know.

God laid out these guidelines clearly.
What is Solomon known for?

Horses and Chariots

Solomon was quite the equestrian. First Kings 4:26–28 (NIV) reads:

> Solomon had four thousand stalls for chariot horses, and twelve thousand horses.

> The district governors, each in his month, supplied provisions for King Solomon and all who came to the king's table. They saw to it that nothing was lacking. They also brought to the proper place their quotas of barley and straw for the chariot horses and the other horses.

This might seem like a noble practice or even a fun hobby for a king, had we not read God's command in Deuteronomy 17.

Wives

Solomon loved his women. Forget God's creation intent, where one man would enjoy one woman for the rest of his life. Solomon wanted more than one . . . more than one hundred, actually.

First Kings 11 provides just a glimpse of the harem that Solomon had going on:

> King Solomon, however, loved many foreign women besides Pharaoh's daughter—Moabites, Ammonites, Edomites, Sidonians and Hittites. They were from nations about which the Lord had told the Israelites, "You must not intermarry with them, because they will surely turn your hearts after their gods." Nevertheless, Solomon held fast to them in love. He had seven hundred wives of royal birth and three hundred concubines, and his wives led him astray. As Solomon grew old, his wives turned his heart after other gods, and his heart was not fully devoted to the Lord his God, as the heart of David his father had been. He followed Ashtoreth the goddess of the Sidonians, and Molek the detestable god of the Ammonites.
>
> vv. 1–5 NIV

God knew what he was talking about when he warned Israel about marrying foreign women. And Solomon, in all his wisdom, was no different. His wives convinced him to try worshiping some of their gods. Before he knew it, "his wives turned his heart after other gods."

Funny how God has a reason behind these guidelines. He doesn't just say, "Because I said so!"

Riches

Solomon loved his bling.

First Kings 10 gives us a detailed look:

> The weight of the gold that Solomon received yearly was 666 talents, not including the revenues from merchants and traders and from all the Arabian kings and the governors of the territories.
>
> King Solomon made two hundred large shields of hammered gold. . . .
>
> Then the king made a great throne covered with ivory and overlaid with fine gold. . . . All King Solomon's goblets were gold, and all the household articles in the Palace of the Forest of Lebanon were pure gold. . . . The king had a fleet of trading ships at sea along with the ships of Hiram. Once every three years it returned, carrying gold, silver and ivory, and apes and baboons.
>
> King Solomon was greater in riches and wisdom than all the other kings of the earth.
>
> vv. 14–23 NIV

In short, Solomon didn't listen to any of God's warnings. And what effect did all these horses, women, and riches have on Solomon? First Kings 11:6 sums it up: "So Solomon did evil in the eyes of the Lord; he did not follow the Lord completely, as David his father had done" (NIV).

The story of Solomon is a sad one.

In short, Solomon thought, "Not me. I'm the wisest man who ever lived."

But the truth was, God was right all along. Solomon was vulnerable just like the rest of us. He let the world's lies creep into his life and he eventually turned his back on the Lord.

Boys need to learn that a wise man is a humble man. We are vulnerable to the world's lies. The lies are plenty, and they're powerful. We need to be careful who we surround ourselves with.

We need to teach our young men to surround themselves with people of faith. This doesn't mean they shouldn't befriend nonbelievers; we should always be a light to others. But we need to choose our closest friends wisely. Our inner circle of friends should be people who spur us on to live a life of faith, "as iron sharpens iron" (Proverbs 27:17).

We also need to teach our young men to make good media choices in a world where young people spend so many hours daily with entertainment media and technology. The fact is, study after study reveals that media messages slowly change our thinking. I've cited many of these studies already in this book, like the one from *Psychological Science*, revealing that "Young teens who viewed movies with sexual content were profoundly influenced by what they watched."[4]

What does this mean?

It means we're just like Solomon. If we surround ourselves with the world's philosophies, then we're slowly going to start believing them.

We need to help our young men think twice about the friends they spend the most time with, the lyrics flowing through their headphones, and the images they watch on all their screens.

How can they spot these lies?

One of the best ways to help young people spot lies is to build a solid foundation of truth.

2. A Foundation of Truth

Are you pointing your boys toward the truth?

Let me be a little more specific:

- Are you reading Scripture in the home? (Joshua 1:8)
- Are you modeling what it means to follow Christ? (Psalm 1:1–3)
- Are you making church a priority so each member of your family can fellowship with other believers and hear the truth? (Hebrews 10:25)
- Are you looking for opportunities throughout the day to talk about what God has done? (Deuteronomy 6:5–7)

In a world that is full of explicit lies, we need to teach our boys the explicit truth from God's Word.

I know this sounds cliché, but ask yourself, *Where are my kids hearing the truth?*

If your boy subjects himself to just half the average daily dose of entertainment media and technology, then he's absorbing about five hours a day of TV, music, social media, YouTube, video games . . . the list goes on. And if you want to remind yourself what he's gleaning from those sources, reread chapter 1 in this book, or pop on TheSource4Parents.com and read the last few issues of my Youth Culture Window articles, where I keep you up-to-date with what's trending in the world of youth pop culture.

With this many lies dangling before our kids' eyes and ears . . . *where are they hearing the truth?*

The best place to find truth is straight from the Scriptures. I remember when our family began reading the Bible together after dinner each night. The kids were young and at times it was hard to keep their attention, so we just read it in little bite-sized chunks. I'd read, then I'd ask some big-picture questions about what we learned about God and his people.

If you feel unqualified to talk about the Bible, don't hesitate to buy some devotional resources that teach Scripture in a style that fits your family. I wrote a fictional book titled *The Zombie Apocalypse Survival Guide for Teenagers*. This book follows the lives of three teenagers struggling to survive each day without their parents around to tell them what to do. The tools these teens find the most helpful are a bow and arrow, a crowbar . . . and a Bible. The three of them keep finding themselves in situations where they question, "What's the right thing to do?" The Bible becomes their source of truth in some very tough situations.

I keep getting emails from dads and moms who say, "I can't get my kids to do family devotions, but each night we read a chapter in your *Zombie Survival Guide* and go through the discussion questions and Scripture. They love it."

Kids don't always welcome Bible-reading time. I remember one day when I gathered all my kids together and said, "Okay, we haven't read the Bible in a week, so we're gonna read it together."

They all moaned and kicked their feet in protest.

Funny, I read for about ten minutes and asked some questions about what we read. We ended up having a five-minute discussion. I can't honestly even remember what the discussion was about, but I'll never forget what my daughter Alyssa said when we finished.

"Dad, I never want to read when you say 'let's read the Bible.' But afterwards, I'm always glad we did."

How are our boys going to learn to be men of God if we don't point them to him daily?

Sometimes when we read the truth of God's Word, we're going to encounter the topic of sex, lust, and self-control. Whenever you encounter these passages, you'll notice a common teaching. . . .

3. Knowing When to Flee

My friend Mark Matlock Tweeted the following:

> Parenting is hard. Proactive parenting is harder. Reactive parenting is hardest.[5]

I've never met a parent of teenagers who said, "This parenting thing is a cinch!"

I have met several parents of teens, however, who have said, "I'd like to cinch a rope around my kid's neck if they talk to me like that again!"

My friend Mark is right. Parenting ain't easy. And yes, it takes even more work when you proactively devote yourselves to spending time with your kids, listening to them, getting to know them, and constantly looking for opportunities to talk with them about truth.

But nothing is as difficult, painstaking, and time-consuming as running around after the fact and reacting to the mistakes our kids made.

If only we had taught them how to flee.

We need to teach our boys how to quit flirting with disaster. This topic is so important, I'm devoting an entire chapter to it.

Let's look at what "fleeing" looks like for our sons and daughters.

Fleeing

Knowing when to run

> Flee from sexual immorality. All other sins a person commits are outside the body, but whoever sins sexually, sins against their own body.
>
> 1 Corinthians 6:18 NIV

How can we teach our kids to flee?

Forget our kids for a moment . . . are *we* fleeing sexual temptations?

The Increasingly Difficult Task of Fleeing

Do you ever turn on the TV in a hotel room?

I'm in a hotel room five to ten days a month. If you dare turn on a TV in a hotel today, one of the questions it often asks you, in a sensual voice, is, *"Do you want to watch any adult desires?"*

If you resist that temptation and click to see the main menu with pay-per-view options, it often lists three options: TV, Movies, or Adult Desires.

If you ignore that temptation again and click Movies, then it gives you several options: Still in Theatres, New Releases, Adult Desires.

Do you have the strength to ignore it a third time?

Sometimes I bail out on the pay-per-view all together and just start flipping through the TV channels. Of course, most hotels include HBO or Showtime, so channel flipping can often land you in the middle of a sex scene on one of those channels. Now a man has to make a very tough decision. Are you going to kick the two naked women fondling each other out of your hotel room? This isn't even a question of, "Are you going to click on porn?" . . . it's a question of "Are you going to click away from the porn that is already on your screen?"

Sadly, for most men, this is why we shouldn't even turn on the TV in the first place.

Blame it on our nucleus accumbens, often called the reward center of the brain. This is a part of the brain that is stimulated when it sees something it wants like food or sexual images. The nucleus accumbens mediates the release of dopamine, which we already learned feels good. The nucleus accumbens lights up during the perception of pleasant or arousing images. When you spot your favorite kind of cake across the room at a dinner party and feel a rush that you must have it, blame the nucleus accumbens. Similarly, when guys see a Victoria's Secret commercial come on during the football game . . . guess what lights up?

This part of the brain can also be activated by music. So imagine the dopamine release you can get when you're sitting on the couch with your lover, eating a piece of your favorite cake, and your favorite song comes on.

Then the thinking part of the brain kicks in and decides what to do.

Maybe this is why it gets more difficult to say no to porn with each click. Each click is another boost of dopamine, which is like a snort of cocaine, literally. So by three or four clicks . . . how effective is the reasoning part of the brain going to be?

Anyone who has been in this situation understands why Paul uses the word *flee* when talking about the lure of sexual immorality in 1 Corinthians 6. Fleeing sexual temptation might sometimes require dropping everything and running like Joseph when he shed his jacket and barely escaped Potiphar's wife (Genesis 39).

My advice: Flee before the first click . . . *while you still have some brain left*.

In today's sexually charged world, it's good for all believers, regardless of age, to lay down some boundaries, or dare I say fleeing measures. Personally, I never turn on the TV in my hotel without checking the schedule. My wife and I talk openly about fleeing these kinds of temptations. I meet for accountability with a good friend who is a local pastor; we ask each other tough questions regularly.

In a sexually charged world, fleeing has become a discipline we need to teach.

Fleeing is a concept we have already discussed in this book and will again, especially in the next chapter about pornography. So for this chapter I'm going to focus on specific ways we can teach our sons and daughters uniquely to flee.

Let's start with the girls.

Training Our Daughters to Flee

When most of us think about fleeing sexual temptation, males probably come to mind. After all, males have that overwhelming sex drive, and a much greater percentage of them struggle with porn (we'll see the specifics in the next chapter). So it's primarily men who need to flee . . . *right*?

Then how come an increasing number of women are having affairs? When I sat down with one of my good friends, a psychologist who focuses on counseling couples, I asked him what changes he has noticed in the last decade in the area of sexual relationships among couples.

Without hesitation he replied, "The large number of women who are cheating on their spouses."

"Did it used to be just men?" I asked.

"It was overwhelmingly men. But in the last few years, I can't believe how many women are telling me about their infidelity. I think it's about 50/50 now."

The *Journal of Marital and Family Therapy*'s numbers would agree with my friend. In their recent study, 57 percent of men and 54 percent of women admit to committing infidelity in any relationship they've had.[1]

I guess women are vulnerable to temptations as well, even if for different reasons.

Yes, women might not be just like men, but it doesn't mean they don't have a sex drive. God happened to make sex very pleasurable. Not to mention, a natural desire when you love someone. So females can be vulnerable to sexual temptation like males.

But more commonly, girls give sex to get love.

It's sad but true. It's like this:

Guys give love to get sex.

Girls give sex to get love.

Again, this isn't to say that girls don't enjoy sex. Girls often enjoy consensual sex on several levels. But frequently, girls are giving sex because they know that it is what guys want, and from day one, they have been taught that being sexy is an important part of being a woman. Subconsciously, sex fills a need for acceptance.

He wants me. That means he likes me and values me.

If only.

Not to mention, sex triggers dopamine releases, which feel good, and oxytocin, which makes you feel closer to someone. So it's hard to deny the draw of sex to anyone, male or female.

So just like boys, girls can be susceptible to sexual temptation. We need to teach them why sex is worth the wait, as we discussed in chapter 4, and how to avoid "starting the launch sequence" as we discussed in chapter 5.

What does this look like for a teenage girl today?

1. Teach Your Daughters How Guys Think

If we don't educate our girls, they'll often assume guys think and feel just like they do. We need to coach our girls about the mind of guys. Dads can be a big help sharing the male perspective. Let girls know what drives guys. Pause and point out examples when you see them in the media. Educate girls on how visual guys are, which is why you need to . . .

2. Teach Your Daughters How to Dress Modestly

We talked about it in chapter 6, and it's worth mentioning again—specifically because our girls need to realize that when they wear revealing clothes . . . *it drives guys crazy*! Just because a guy is noticing you doesn't mean he likes you. If only we could put hidden microphones in guys' locker rooms and let girls hear the way guys talk about them. Soon girls would know that they are merely objects to many of these guys. Teach your daughter to prove to the world that she is so much more than just a sex object. Her value goes way beyond dressing sexy.

3. Teach Your Daughters to Beware

Sadly, our girls don't realize how dangerous it is to be alone with guys. We need to let our girls know why it's important not to go to a guy's house when his parents are gone, even if it's "just to do homework." We need to teach our daughters that most teen guys can't give a backrub without secretly wishing they could be touching much more than their back! If guys really care about our girls and not just about sex, then they won't mind hanging out with our girls in public.

Our girls will never learn the truth from today's movies, sitcoms, and music. We need to teach them. We need to teach our girls to flee temptation. Much of this can be done by teaching them how to think through consequences of choices . . . *even unintended consequences.*

Unintended Consequences

The Center of Alcohol Studies at Rutgers University tackled a research project (posted in *The Journal of Studies on Alcohol and Drugs*), in which they followed hundreds of young women from their senior year in high school through their freshman year of college. The study found two alarming discoveries:

- "Of women who had never drunk heavily in high school (if at all), nearly half admitted to binge drinking at least once by the end of their first college semester."
- "Of all young women whose biggest binge had included four to six drinks, one quarter said they'd been sexually victimized in the fall semester. That included anything from unwanted sexual contact to rape. And the more alcohol those binges involved, the greater the likelihood of sexual assault. Of women who'd ever consumed 10 or more drinks in a sitting since starting college, 59% were sexually victimized by the end of their first semester."[2]

It's alarming to discover that almost half of female college freshmen exercised their newfound freedom by engaging in a very risky behavior. Binge drinking is no joke. It's not just having a beer or a glass of wine. Binge drinking is drinking to get drunk.

This isn't surprising, considering the media messages young people see and hear every day. Teenagers are bombarded with the "drink it up" and "raise your glass" messages from almost every entertainment media source.

But how many consequences do these sources show?

When is the last time you saw the star of your teen's favorite sitcom get raped or sexually victimized?

The consequences many of the girls in this study endured is even more terrifying. Rape or sexual victimization is a nightmare and often life changing. And to think that anywhere from 25 to 59 percent of these women experienced this as a result of their binge is sobering. Literally.

Are you talking with your daughter about these kinds of decisions and unintended consequences?

How can someone flee when they're drunk or passed out?

But these kinds of tragedies don't only occur when alcohol is involved. Sometimes girls put themselves in danger even when they have all their inhibitions.

Years ago I took a group of several hundred middle school students on a weekend trip to the beach. For safety, we required the kids to stay in groups. I did this trip for almost a decade without a hitch. Then one year . . . *catastrophe struck.*

It was almost bedtime, and one of my female leaders approached me, visibly shaken. "Jonathan, I need to talk with you."

We stepped away from the crowd and I asked her what was wrong.

"I don't even know how to say this," she said. She looked like she had seen a ghost.

"What's wrong?"

"It's 'Vanessa.' She's bleeding . . . from her vagina."

I tried not to be condescending. "Uh, this happens, as you know, girls go through—"

"It's not her period," she interrupted. "She was raped. Well . . . I don't know what you call it. He used his hand and he forced himself in her."

It's called *digital rape*, so we discovered about an hour later as we were filling out the police report. Vanessa had met a guy on the boardwalk and got some friends to cover for her while she went off with him. They lay down in a private grassy area secluded by the cliffs.

They were making out for only a minute or so before this young man started moving his hand up her shirt. She had never let a guy do that before, but she didn't stop him. She later admitted she wanted him to like her.

Soon he began moving his hand up her leg. She pushed his hand away and said no. He stopped for a moment but then his hand found its way back to her leg again.

She tried to stop his hand several times but he soon pinned both her hands down with his left hand so he was free to use his right hand as he wished. He kept telling her, "Shut up. I know you want it."

She cried the entire time.

I had to call her father and let him know what happened to his baby girl.

Rape isn't sex. It's an act of violence. Nothing Vanessa did deserved the unplanned consequences she received. But she and her friends made a foolish choice thinking it was not only romantic but safe to wander off alone with a cute guy. Even cute guys can be rapists. Vanessa learned that the hard way.

We need to teach our daughters about predators. We need to teach them not to get alone with any guy. He could be a great guy who is just struggling with sexual temptation, or he could be a predator, but our daughters shouldn't be alone with either guy.

After twenty years of studying youth culture and hanging out with teenagers, here's what I've observed about young girls today:

They know enough about being sexy to attract guys . . .
but not enough to beware.

Are you ready to have these conversations with your daughter?

Training Our Sons to Flee

"Stephen" never wanted to be a slave to his desires, but it was only a matter of a few weeks and he couldn't stop on his own power. It was only when his parents discovered his habit that he was prompted to stop.

That's when I met him. His dad called me and asked if I'd talk with him. I knew the teen from church, and he wanted to talk with me.

A few days later we were sitting together at a nearby hamburger joint, dipping our fries in ketchup and talking about football.

The conversation paused and I finally asked him, "Why did you want to talk with me?"

His posture changed. This cool, confident kid began hunching in his chair. His shoulders dropped and he looked down at his plate.

"I found some pictures online," he began. "I was in the den one night—that's where we keep our computer—and I can't even remember how I got there, but I saw some pictures that I knew I wasn't supposed to be looking at. But I clicked anyway."

He paused and took a sip of his Coke. "The next day I couldn't get those pictures out of my head, so that night, when my parents went to bed, I snuck into the den and found them again. This time I looked at even more pictures."

"What did you think?" I asked.

He shrugged his shoulders. "I dunno. I liked them, I guess," he answered honestly.

"So night after night I'd sneak into the den when my parents were away or asleep, and I'd look at pictures."

"How long did this go on?" I asked.

He looked up and shrugged his shoulders again. "I dunno. Maybe a couple weeks.

"Then one night I was clicking around and everywhere I went it kept saying, *Enter your card number and you can see everything*. I didn't have a card." He paused and looked up at me. "But my mom did."

"So what did you do?" I asked.

"I snuck into my mom's room, quietly grabbed her wallet out of her purse, and took her credit card."

"Then what happened?"

His eyes got big and he exhaled. "I saw *everything*!"

"Was it what you hoped for?" I inquired.

He thought for a minute, chewing on his lower lip. "Not really. I pretty much just wondered, *what's next*?"

"So why are we here?" I asked.

He snorted. "Because my mom just got her credit card bill."

Stephen's story rings true with many today, except that most don't use credit cards and many don't get caught. But as you'll find out in the next chapter, millions upon millions of young boys navigate porn sites regularly. Well over half of teenage boys.

Sexual temptation is a huge lure for young men. Whether it's porn, masturbation, hooking up for casual sex, or the pressure they feel when they get alone with their girlfriends, today's young men feel enticed by sexual temptation recurrently.

It's not a surprise with the abundance of sexually charged images and messages bombarding them daily, if not hourly. Young people today are inundated with stimuli encouraging them to think sexual thoughts and act out in some way.

In the next two chapters I'll talk specifically about pornography and masturbation, and how to flee those temptations. So for this chapter, let's focus on teaching our boys to flee sexual temptation with the girls they encounter day to day.

The Bible tells us to flee youthful lusts (2 Timothy 2:22) and specifically sexual temptation (1 Corinthians 6:18). What does this look like each day for our sons?

1. Teach Your Son Not to Turn His Head

It happens like this: A pretty girl walks by. What do most guys do? They turn their heads and take a closer look (and they usually aren't checking out her hairstyle). I told my son, "Don't feel guilty if you notice a pretty girl . . . but leave it at that. When you turn for that second look, it's usually lusting."

2. Teach Your Son to Browse Publicly

Doctors recommend parents shouldn't allow computers or smartphones in their kids' bedrooms. Instead, they say put a computer in a family area and monitor their computer use. Why? Probably because they know the temptations that private late-night browsing can cause. We should teach our kids not to put themselves in tempting situations. Browsing an unmonitored computer with no one around is a good way to open yourself up to temptation, and it's what leads the majority of men in this country to look at porn.

3. Teach Your Son Not to Get Alone With a Girl

Every bit of entertainment we watch seems to sell us on the fact that men should always invite a girl in or park with her on a dark road or a secluded hilltop overlooking the city. If you follow situations like these to their natural conclusion, sex is the result. We can't just teach our kids God's design for sex; we also need to teach our boys how to avoid "initiating the launch sequence." Getting alone with a girl is flirting with disaster.

4. Teach Your Son to Talk About It

The Bible encourages us to "confess our sins to each other" so we can be healed (James 5:16). We need to teach our boys to find mentors and friends who can hold them accountable. This is where plugging in to a church can really help. Most youth pastors are recruiting teams of volunteers who are willing to be a voice of counsel and encouragement in the lives of our kids. Help your boy seek out positive male role models in his life whom he can talk to and share real-life struggles. Yes, parents can act in this role, but encourage your kids to connect with other positive adult role models too.

Where We Are Running

Sometimes we can be so focused on running away, we never ask, "What are we running toward?"

One of the best passages in the Bible equipping us to flee sin is a passage that isn't about fleeing. It's about where we should be focusing:

> Therefore, since we are surrounded by such a huge crowd of witnesses to the life of faith, let us strip off every weight that slows us down, especially the sin that so easily trips us up. And let us run with endurance the race God has set before us. We do this by keeping our eyes on Jesus, the champion who initiates and perfects our faith. Because of the joy awaiting him, he endured the cross, disregarding its shame. Now he is seated in the place of honor beside God's throne.
>
> Hebrews 12:1–2

Where are your eyes fixed?

What a great passage to discuss with your kids. Read this and ask them:

- What are some of the weights that slow us down?
- What are some weights that you might need to strip off?
- Where does this Scripture tell us to fix our eyes?
- How can we fix our eyes on Jesus today, this week, this month?

My brother Thom is a pastor, and recently he told the story of how he met his wife, Amy. Thom had been living for himself for a few years, pursuing all kinds of temporary thrills that life offers. All this time, he was hoping he'd find a girl that was "the one." No one really fit the mold.

After quite a while of doing things his way, he met a friend who encouraged him to start pursuing God. Thom not only began fleeing his old temptations, he began running toward positive activities for the first time in a long time. He began going to church and even volunteered in ministry occasionally.

Seeing his change of heart, I invited him to come help me on a one-day ministry trip. It was there that he met a really pretty Christian girl named Amy, who was one of my volunteers.

The rest is history.

When Thom started pursuing God, other areas of his life began falling into place.

Resisting temptation isn't just about running away. It's about what we should be running toward.

What is your family running toward?

We can help our kids pursue good things and live life to the full (John 10:10)!

Paul warns us about a lot of sins in the New Testament: gossip, anger, bitterness, stealing, drunkenness, even acting generally foolish. But there's only one sin that he literally instructs us to run away from.

Do you think we should listen?

Well, most people don't, as we'll see in the next chapter.

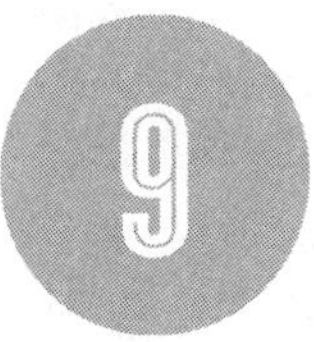

The Lure of Porn

From **Game of Thrones** to hard-core addictions

"It's hilarious. Just search for it on Google Images."

That's how it started.

"Chris" was only twelve years old when his friend told him about the funny meme, those popular Internet pictures with humorous captions. But what started as an innocent search quickly led down a rabbit trail to hard-core porn.

Chris had actually never stumbled on any pornographic images before, probably because his parents had tried to be really careful. They didn't have porn filters on the family computer, but it was at a desk in the great room, right next to the TV and the kitchen, and Mom or Dad were always right there when Chris browsed the web. Chris's parents didn't allow his phone or the family iPad in the bedroom. Plus, they set some parental restrictions on those mobile devices to prevent access to most sexual content.

But this particular afternoon, Chris's dad was still at work and his mom was running errands. Chris didn't think anything about booting up the computer alone in the house. He had done it before.

And today he was simply curious about the funny picture his friend had described.

A quick click of the mouse, a few taps of his fingers on the keyboard, and he was browsing through Google images looking for the funny meme.

In the third row of pictures, second from the right, a girl wearing a bikini appeared. The caption was enticing.

Chris's heart rate accelerated and he shifted in the squeaky computer chair. He looked over his shoulder. No one was there. He knew that, but couldn't help but double-check.

He slowly scrolled the cursor over to the right, landing on the picture of the girl. A quick click and he was looking at the image full size. A button invited him to visit the page the picture originated from.

He stared at the picture for a moment, taking it all in. He had seen pictures of girls in bikinis before, but they had only really started to interest him in the last year. Plus, this girl was truly mesmerizing. Her bikini top barely covered all she had—and she had plenty. Her smile was enticing, especially the way she was licking her lips ever so slightly.

Chris didn't wait another second. He clicked VISIT PAGE.

One click led to another, and less than five minutes later Chris was watching a video of two Ukrainian girls doing things he had never even dreamed about. It was his first exposure to hard-core pornography; actually, his first time exposed to porn of any kind.

Could Chris's parents have done more? Maybe.

Did they do anything wrong? It's hard to cast stones. We live in a world where porn is literally seeping through every digital and analog signal crawling through our homes. Sometimes it's difficult to keep up.

What can caring parents do?

First Exposure

I'll never forget my first exposure to porn. My family was visiting another family from our church. They had two boys close to the same age as my brother and me. The adults assembled in the living room, drinking coffee and discussing boring grown-up matters, while the kids quickly retreated to the backyard to climb trees, dig holes, and hit each other with sticks.

It was only a matter of minutes before the older brother—I can't remember his name—looked over his shoulder and then whispered to us, "Do you want to see something?"

We followed him to an alley behind his house. He moved a few bricks in the back of a junk pile, revealing a magazine. I can't remember the title, but I remember the pictures well. The first picture I saw was of a completely naked woman spreading her legs, revealing something I had only seen as sketch drawings in an illustrated picture book about the human body. But what I was seeing in this magazine was so vivid, so captivating . . . I couldn't look away as he flipped from page to page.

I honestly can't tell you if I was turned on or just fascinated. But I know I liked what I saw.

I was nine years old.

I saw a handful of other magazines in the next few years, at school, at a friend's house, a sneak peek in a neighborhood convenience store . . . I wasn't addicted, but I never turned down a free glimpse. At twelve years old my neighborhood friend showed me his dad's *Penthouse* magazine. I looked at it for literally hours, reading some of the stories and digesting each picture again and again. I had never seen pictures like these for more than a few seconds. My friend's parents weren't going to be home for a while. I had plenty of time to take it all in.

I can still recall many of those images from that magazine. In fact, later that night the images haunted me so greatly, I was plagued with guilt and ended up confessing everything to my dad.

My friend found out the next day and called me a wimp. (He actually used another word.)

A year later I was at the same friend's house and he pulled a VHS tape off the shelf with the label *Tora! Tora! Tora!* With a smirk on his face he asked, "Do you want to see something?" I had a feeling we weren't going to watch *Tora! Tora! Tora!*

Moments later we were watching hard-core porn. This was thirty years ago, and I can still tell you explicit details of this film. I remember the title, and I remember the name of the female porn star. I got to know her well in the next few months, because every chance I had, I was at my friend's house watching the tape labeled "*Tora! Tora! Tora!*" over and over again.

I learned a lot about human anatomy from that ninety-minute film, and even more about the lure of sexual temptation.

That was 1984, before the Internet.

I can't imagine the temptation young people endure today.

As I reflect back on this experience, I remember being magnetically drawn to the visuals of this film. I couldn't get enough of it. It was the most arousing feeling I had ever experienced. That's probably why I always disappeared to the bathroom immediately after the film to do what most young boys do when they crave sexual release.

Then the guilt would kick in.

Then one day my friend's dad randomly decided he wanted to watch *Tora! Tora! Tora!* . . . and that was the end of that.

Today Porn Is Everywhere

In my world, it wasn't easy to find porn. I had to search for it and then sneak behind the backs of adults to watch it. With the exception of my *Tora! Tora! Tora!* binge, it probably only happened a couple times a year. If I had been offered an avenue to see more, I'm embarrassed to admit, I might have traveled that road every day, perhaps multiple times.

Today porn bombards us through every cable and signal permeating our homes. Unless we all shut off the power grid and move to a shack in the mountains, porn is readily accessible.

If you have the Internet, the most explicit and depraved forms of porn are just a click away. If you ever stay in a hotel, hard-core porn is always one of the TV's main menu choices. If you're like the 91 percent of Americans who pay for TV reception at home, adult channels and pay-per-view porn are available at the click of your remote, not to mention the soft-core porn that they often show for free on Cinemax, Showtime, and HBO.

Maybe that's why 87 percent of men admitted to using porn in the past year. If that weren't enough, 69 percent of men and 10 percent of women report viewing pornography more than once a month.[1]

The U.S. has pandemic porn problems:

- Every year, pornography generates $13 billion in the U.S.
- Twenty-four percent of smartphone owners admit to having pornographic material on their mobile devices.
- Fifty percent of all Christian men and 20 percent of all Christian women say they are addicted to pornography.[2]

Sadly, when you look at the porn habits of teenagers, the numbers aren't any prettier:

- Ninety-three percent of boys and 62 percent of girls are exposed to porn before their eighteenth birthday.[3]
- Seventy-one percent of teenagers feel the need to hide their online activity from parents.[4]
- Fifteen percent of boys and 9 percent of girls have viewed (illegal) child pornography online.[5]

If your kids are eleven or older, chances are they have already stumbled upon it at least once.

Numbers can be scary . . . and frankly, you'll see a lot of numbers thrown around in today's parenting articles and blogs, varying in results. Sometimes it's hard to determine which numbers are correct.

But I'm sure no one would argue with this: Porn is way too convenient and available to our kids today.

The important question is, how should we respond?

Inside the World of Porn

Parents know porn exists, and as much as we would like to deny it, we know it's a viable threat to our kids. That's probably why I hear the same question, almost verbatim, at almost every one of my parent workshops:

> *"What can we do to keep our kids from accessing inappropriate material?"*

That's what I asked my friend Craig Gross. Craig is the founder of XXXchurch.com, a ministry assisting people who are struggling with pornography addiction. Craig and his ministry have spent the last decade developing tools to help people young and old, both male and female, escape the bondage of pornography.

Craig is a dad traversing the same real-life issues the rest of us are navigating daily.

After catching up a little bit, I dove right into the subject at hand, asking Craig about the first age of porn exposure. "I've heard tons of different statistics thrown around," I disclosed. "Which ones should we believe?"

"Eleven years old," Craig answered. "That seems to be when most kids first stumble upon porn. But many discover it before then. I think it's good to start talking with your kids about sex when they are about seven or eight."

I pushed back just a little. "But what about that parent who thinks, *Not my kid. My kid isn't interested in that stuff*?"

Craig chuckled. "Many parents think, *Not my kid.* Those are frequently the parents who end up contacting our ministry a year later and begging us to solve their problems, because now their kid is addicted to porn."

"So what's the best advice you can give to parents about keeping their kids safe from the lure of pornography?" I asked.

Craig didn't hesitate for even a second. "Be proactive. Most parents are reactive instead of proactive. They wait until porn has infiltrated their house, then they go around trying to put out the fires."

"So how can parents be proactive?"

"First, talk with your kids about it," Craig responded matter-of-factly. "Don't be afraid to tell them the truth."

"What can parents say?" I inquired.

"Don't just say *no*, say *why*."

"So if your son wants to spend time talking with strangers on the social media site Omegle, dialogue with him about the kind of content he'll encounter?"

"Exactly. Don't leave them with, 'Because I said so.'"

"What if our kids sneak and go to racy sites when we're not there?" I proposed.

"That is why it's also important for families to put up some safeguards in the home."

"What kind of safeguards do you use?"

"I just bought this Skydog router, and I use X3watch."

A router is the little box that acts as the distribution center for the home's Internet, both Wi-Fi and what is plugged into your computer. Any home with Wi-Fi has one.

"Tell me more about those safeguards," I said.

"The router allows me to block out some sites at the router level. This makes me feel a little better about my kids' friends using our Wi-Fi. The X3 software is something we at XXXchurch.com offer. It helps parents know where their kids are navigating on the web."

(Craig's ministry is great at providing software solutions to help parents battle the lure of pornography in the home. Jump on XXXchurch.com to see their most current software.)

"Is this just a problem with young men, Craig?"

"Sadly, no. Forty percent of porn visitors are female."

"In all honesty," I interjected, "do you think girls are as interested in porn as the guys?"

"Well, forty-eight percent of the people attending porn shows are women. Guys bring them. Girls know it's what their boyfriend wants, so they are complying."

Three Parenting Practices Preventing the Permeation of Porn

Parents are looking for practical ways to battle the threat of porn in their home. Of all the research and advice available on the subject today, here are the three common truths I see over and over again . . .

1. Don't Underestimate the Power of Porn

We need to understand the power and pervasiveness of porn. If you've forgotten how readily available sexual content is in our world today, I encourage you to reread chapter 1 in this book. I can honestly tell you that you can't protect your kids from it.

Don't get me wrong, I'm not saying all our kids are going to become porn addicts. And more important, I'm not saying to just give up. I'm trying to remind you that unless you literally lock your kids in the basement and never let them go outside or turn on any entertainment media . . . your kids are going to be exposed to some sexual content.

If your kids watch TV, they will hear sexual references, jokes, and innuendos frequently.

As I write this, *Family Guy* is still one of the most popular shows watched by young people. Have you ever watched an episode of *Family Guy*? I know families who let their ten-year-olds watch the show. Are you ready to explain what fellatio is when your ten-year-old hears it mentioned on the show?

In 2014, *The Voice* was in the top ten on the Nielsen charts almost any given week of the season. Shakira's stardom increased tenfold during her season as a judge, so it wasn't surprising when her hit song "Can't Remember to Forget You" was in the top 100 of the music and music-video charts for much of the year. In this video, Shakira sang nearly naked or in lingerie before ending up on a bed with Rihanna as they groped themselves and each other. Even *Elle* magazine referred to "all the ridiculously hot, nearly naked looks from Shakira and Rihanna's new video."[6]

And this is just what kids are gleaning from the "clean" programming our world offers.

Entertainment media is only becoming more loaded with sexual content and images. Millennial experts Ypulse named *Game of Thrones* the most popular show watched by college kids. I already talked about the show in chapter 1, but let me just reiterate: This show is ridiculously pornographic. The only difference between *Game of Thrones* sex scenes and hard-core porn sex scenes are extreme closeup shots.

It doesn't take an expert to realize that all these sexual messages and images make kids even more curious about something that is already enticing.

So where do they go for answers?

"Google is the new sex ed." I'm starting to hear that phrase more frequently.

Anne Marie Miller is the first person I heard use this phrase in her article "3 Things You Don't Know About Your Children and Sex." After spending a summer speaking to kids about sex and counseling them, she kept hearing the same thing over and over again. Whenever she inquired about a young person's first exposure to pornography, she heard the same answer—*Google Image searching.*[7]

Kids are going to the web, rather than parents, for their answers for two reasons:

- **It's the place they go for answers about everything else.** How tall is the Golden Gate Bridge? Google it. How many sizes of poodles are there, anyway? Google it. What is anal sex? Google it.
- **Sex is an embarrassing subject, so kids would rather ask questions anonymously.** Experts are noticing a growing trend in the popularity of anonymous websites. Young people have learned that the content they post on the most popular social media sites is scrutinized by parents, bosses, and enemies. Hence the rise in "anonymous" social media apps and websites. It's easier to talk about embarrassing subjects when no one knows who you are. *The Washington Post* asserts, "Anonymous and ephemeral, apps such as Whisper, Secret, Ask.fm and Snapchat fill a growing demand among teens for more fun, less accountability and more privacy online."[8] Young people are getting used to anonymity. It's no surprise when they go online instead of face-to-face for their answers to embarrassing questions. They love the lack of accountability.

The presence of porn is only growing more pervasive.

Just because our boys are more commonly affected by the visuals of porn, it doesn't mean our daughters are immune from it. I constantly encounter youth workers who are counseling girls addicted to porn, but even more frequently, I hear about girls who are giving in to guys' expectations driven by porn.

Author Penny Marshall wrote about this trend, interviewing girls in their young teens complaining about their boyfriends pressuring them to dress like porn stars, wear sexy underwear, have bodies like porn stars, and "behave like them when we are alone."

In her research, she met a sixteen-year-old girl who had been dating a boy for four months, and liked him, but was scared by him whenever they got alone because, she claimed, "He changes."

> Suddenly, when we are being intimate, he'll say something that he must have heard in a porn film. For example, he'll call me a "bitch" and use dirty language that he'd never use normally. It's awful. It's so obvious he's copying his actions from watching porn. No boy would call you beautiful. They use words like "hot" and "sexy." . . . It's all about performing sexual acts for them, and they assume we'll love it.[9]

Parents need to stop deceiving themselves. We live in a sexually charged world, and chances are your kids are stumbling upon sexually charged messages and images frequently. If you want to battle the threat of porn in your home, start by opening your eyes to the reality of the situation. Porn is powerful, pervasive, and permeating.

That's why we need to open up the doors of communication about it in our homes.

2. Look for Opportunities to Dialogue About Porn

It's the one solution everybody, and I mean *everybody* agrees on.

I've been researching youth culture, studying parenting practices, and teaching parent workshops for over a decade now. I've read countless studies speculating how to be a better parent, how to reduce the risk of pregnancy and STDs, how to steer kids away from drugs and alcohol . . . I've read it all. And the one deduction

I can wholeheartedly conclude is . . . *no one agrees!* I've read reputable studies that say more boundaries are the answer, where other respectable studies conclude the exact opposite—more freedom is just what kids need. But in all the studies, from all the PhDs in every university and practice imaginable, one common theme emerges. Every single expert agrees: *We need to talk with our kids about this all the time.*

And sadly . . . it's the one thing parents don't do.

So how do we have this conversation?

First, remember a principle that I keep repeating throughout this book. It's not one conversation—it's many. Look for opportunities to have these conversations. If a favorite TV character decides to sleep with his girlfriend, hit the Pause button and talk about it. Bring it up at dinner and ask their opinion. Do more listening than lecturing. More dialogue than monologue.

If the only time we dialogue with our kids is when we want to teach them something, we're missing the point. We should be talking with our kids about everything. If you notice your five-year-old carrying around a particular teddy bear, ask him about it.

Why?

Because as parents we love our kids and want to get to know them better. Even the names of their teddy bears.

"Who's that?"

"It's Rufus."

"Tell me about Rufus."

The more we listen to our kids in daily life, the more they'll come to us when they really need someone to listen.

As they grow and become more curious about sex, it won't be a surprise when we discuss it with them. After all . . . we talk about everything.

Don't be afraid to use discussion tools. My last book, *Get Your Teenager Talking*, is full of discussion questions that open doors to meaningful conversations. Crack a book like that open at dinner and ask your kids what they think about real-life issues.

Dads, don't be afraid to meet with your sons once a week for breakfast and go through a devotional that speaks candidly about these issues. My devotional, *The Guy's Guide to God, Girls, and the Phone in Your Pocket*, has been called "refreshingly brutal." It gives advice like, "If you have to look over your shoulder to check if anyone's in the room, you probably shouldn't be typing it into the search engine," or, "God wants you to enjoy a naked woman . . . *one* naked woman." The book has countless entries about sex, temptation, and the way we should treat the opposite sex.

Books can be great resources, but don't hesitate to use your Bible as well. Share Scripture and ask questions about what you read. Start with 2 Timothy 2:22 and 1 Corinthians 6:18.

Use questions as often as possible. Constantly look for any opportunity to listen to your kids' hearts about the issues they are struggling with.

But let's not forget to create an environment where our kids can learn to make these decisions without being bombarded with sexual content at every turn.

3. Place Safeguards

No, we can't protect our kids from everything. And frankly, I don't think we should try to remove our kids from every danger. If we swoop down and save our kids from every tough decision they have to make, how can we expect them to learn how to make decisions?

But that doesn't mean we should raise our kids in the red-light district.

This is a tough balance at times.

I recommend setting some realistic and fair safeguards in the home, especially while the kids are younger. And I don't mean just porn blocks. Today's kids need boundaries in numerous areas of entertainment media and technology. I recommend frequent conversations about being wise with media, and boundaries that hold our kids accountable to that wisdom.

Doctor's orders.

Seriously. Doctors frequently release studies about the effects of entertainment media on young people. For example, the American Academy of Pediatrics recently published a report titled "Children, Adolescents and the Media," unveiling the effects of media on children zero to seventeen years old. These doctors recommended the following to parents:

- Limit the amount of total entertainment screen time to less than two hours per day.
- Discourage screen media exposure for children less than two years of age.
- Keep the TV and Internet-connected electronic devices out of the child's bedroom.
- Monitor what media your children are using and accessing, including any websites they are visiting and social media sites they may be using.
- Co-view TV, movies, and videos with children and teenagers, and use this as a way of discussing important family values.
- Model active parenting by establishing a family home use plan for all media. As part of the plan, enforce a bedtime "curfew" for media devices, including cell phones. Establish reasonable but firm rules about cell phones, texting, Internet, and social media use.[10]

Note: This report wasn't from Focus on the Family or some Christian publication. This is what secular doctors are recommending.

Are you teaching your kids how to make responsible decisions about entertainment media and technology?

Do you know what apps your kids are using? Do you "co-view" TV shows, movies, and YouTube videos with your kids? Have you had conversations about who they are communicating with in social media? Have you set some helpful guidelines and curfews for the entertainment media and technology in your house?

This is what these pediatricians recommend.

Don't feel pressured to buy your ten-year-old a phone or a tablet just because every one of her friends has one. You're not doing your kids a favor if you let YouTube, TV, and social media raise your kids.

When my kids were younger, we set some pretty strict guidelines to help them see the truth through the dense fog of entertainment lies. As they turned fifteen and sixteen, we lightened up a little, allowing them to make more decisions, but we kept some helpful guidelines:

- Phone off at night.
- Tuesday night—no entertainment media. We read and play games as a family.
- Mom and Dad have all passwords and can look at your phone whenever they want.

These rules didn't hinder them from learning to make good media decisions themselves. On the contrary, they taught them discipline and restraint. My older daughter, now off at college, says she wishes we could have had more nights of "no entertainment media."

Entertainment media is full of lies. Guidelines, passwords, and porn blocks keep all our kids from encountering distractions at every click of a button.

I realize that porn filters aren't foolproof. That's why I wrote about the importance of having frequent conversations before writing about safeguards. Some people subscribe to some sort of "Net Nanny" and think they're done raising their kids. Porn blocks aren't the answer; they just help our kids see through the sexually charged fog that permeates much of the world wide web today.

What porn blocks work best? The second I write about it, it will become outdated, so I recommend going to the place our kids go for answers: Google. Do a quick Google search for "porn blocks" or "porn filters." You'll see advertisements for hardware and software, and you'll also see articles with advice and reviews about which blocks work best. Do a little research. Ask fellow parents what they use. Jump on XXXchurch.com and see the articles and software they offer.

Just realize, porn filters aren't going to block out Shakira nearly naked on YouTube, and you'll find that some porn can slip through—hence the need for continual conversations. But these kinds of safeguards can help your kids browse the web without being bombarded at every turn.

In addition to porn filters, investigate how to use parental controls on your kids' phones and other mobile devices. When they're young, use a high amount of control, blocking out anything questionable. You have the password and only you download new apps. As they get older, give them more control as they prove themselves trustworthy, but continue to hold them accountable. In other words, maybe give your kids the ability to download apps themselves, but ask them about the apps frequently and have them show you what they do. Ask them what their experience has been. Teach them to make good media decisions—after all, when they turn eighteen and are on their own . . . they can download whatever they want.

Are you equipping them for that day?

If you'd like to know more about this, I write about parenting, youth culture, entertainment media, and technology constantly in my articles and blog on TheSource4Parents.com.

What If I Discover My Kid Viewing Porn?

Sadly, many of our kids will discover porn. Sometimes they'll tell us, but many times they won't.

If you discover your kids looking at porn, consider these three steps:

1. Sleep on Your Response

As parents, our first reaction can often be overreaction.

Suppress the temptation to handle it right then. *Very few* parents handle these situations well on the fly. Buy yourself some time and say something like this:

> We just discovered what you have been looking at on your computer/phone/mobile device. I'm not exactly sure what is best to do at the moment, so we want to wait, pray, and sleep on the decision. In the meantime, I want you to go unplug/power-down your computer/phone/mobile device and keep it off for the next twenty-four hours until we talk tomorrow. We love you so much, this is too important for us to overreact and do something hasty and brash.

This accomplishes two tasks: (1) It truly buys you time to think, pray, and sleep on your decision. I find that wisdom sometimes comes in a slow trickle, where ignorance expels like a fire hose; and (2) the wait will give them time to think about what they did. Sometimes that is a punishment in itself.

Many kids might even say, "No, I want to deal with this now!" The wait will be torturous. If this is the case, and if you have the self-control to restrain your reaction, then tell them:

> You can feel free to talk with us. We're always here to listen to you. We just want to withhold making any decisions tonight. So feel free to share anything you like with us. We welcome it. Just please don't expect us to resolve something tonight. We need time.

After buying some time . . .

2. Seek to Understand

Start by trying to understand the situation. Ask them questions because you care, not because you're trying to dig up incriminating evidence.

Here are some questions you might use:

- When did this start and how did it progress?
- How did this make you feel?
- Did you ever tell anyone? Did this person help the situation?
- Do you think there are any natural consequences that you might experience from this situation?
- What would you do if you could do this all over again?
- How do you think we should respond?

In some cases, boys might be more comfortable talking with just Dad about this, and girls with Mom . . . but not always. In some situations it might not be bad to have both parents giving assurance of their love. Consider what would make it easiest for your kids to open up.

Let your kids see your love and grace throughout this process. As you listen and seek to understand them, you might even be able to share some stories from your own life of overcoming struggles and temptations. Remember to listen more than you lecture, though. Focus on helping them feel heard and understood.

3. Propose a Plan of Purity

Jesus had an amazing way with sinners.

As a sinner, I can't help but be attracted to it. In fact, the more sinful a person was in the Gospel accounts, the more they seemed to want to be near Jesus. It's almost as if people wanted freedom from the bondage of their sin, and cherished the opportunity to encounter someone who would not only respond in love and grace, but offer deliverance.

Think about it: Zacchaeus (Luke 19), the woman at the well (John 4), the woman caught in adultery (John 8), the sinful woman who anointed Jesus' feet (Luke 7) . . . Jesus didn't dwell on their sinful pasts; instead, he provided grace and a fresh start for their future.

How can we help give our kids a fresh start for the future?

Many might instinctively think *punishment*.

I think we should consider *deliverance*.

If you catch your kids looking at naked pictures, confront them, sleep on it for twenty-four hours, then trudge through the whole scenario with them. . . . That whole experience is almost a punishment itself. The shame of being caught by Mom and/or Dad was no doubt one of the most embarrassing and humbling moments ever experienced. My guess is . . . *Johnny doesn't need a spanking too*.

Instead, come up with a plan for deliverance and healing.

A. Make Sure They Understand the Truth About Sex

We've been talking about God's gift of sex throughout this whole book, but specifically in chapter 4, "The Most Enjoyable Sex." Help them understand that lusting after pornographic pictures is wrong and God can deliver them from that bondage.

Share some of the truth I've been highlighting in this book. If I caught my son looking at porn, I might say:

Son, I totally understand the temptation you're experiencing. In fact, it's a common temptation all men have; you're not alone. The reason why you want to look at a naked woman is because God created you to enjoy looking at a naked woman . . . *one* naked woman. Take a look at Proverbs 5:18–23 with me.

> Let your wife be a fountain of blessing for you.
> Rejoice in the wife of your youth.
> She is a loving deer, a graceful doe.
> Let her breasts satisfy you always.
> May you always be captivated by her love.

Then I might ask:

- Who does God say is a blessing for us?
- What should we let satisfy us always?

But then keep reading:

> Why be captivated, my son, by an immoral woman,
> or fondle the breasts of a promiscuous woman?
> For the Lord sees clearly what a man does,
> examining every path he takes.
> An evil man is held captive by his own sins;
> they are ropes that catch and hold him.
> He will die for lack of self-control;
> he will be lost because of his great foolishness.

Then I'd ask:

- Who should we not be captivated by or attracted to?
- Whose breasts aren't for us?
- Where are some places we might encounter these kinds of distractions today, the breasts of women who aren't our wives?
- What are some of the "ropes that catch and hold" us?
- What will happen to us if we lack self-control?

Help your kids understand that God wants them to enjoy sex with their spouses someday, but the gift of sex was created to be shared between one man and one woman. Just like sleeping with someone before you're married lingers into marriage, porn brings others into the marriage bed. Porn becomes a rope or snare that catches us and holds us captive from the freedom God provides in our lives.

Talk about lust. Help your kids understand the pitfalls of lusting and how to escape it. (We go over this in detail in the next chapter, about masturbation.)

The world is full of messages that say, "Just lose control" or "Do what feels right at the moment." The Bible tells us to give God control.

B. Help Them Recognize Natural Consequences

If your son is the one caught viewing porn, let him know some of the natural consequences, like impotence. This isn't a scare tactic; it's just the truth. The fact is, impotence is increasing, and many men are not satisfied with their sexual partner (I'd love to say "wife" here, but unfortunately, for many it's just "sexual partner") because they're truly becoming addicted to the never-ending stream of dopamine spikes they get from watching different women do different things at the click of a button.[11]

The more porn guys watch, the more difficult it is to become turned on. This is becoming a huge problem with young men, *Psychology Today* explains:

> Desperate young men from various cultures, with different levels of education, religiosity, attitudes, values, diets, marijuana use and personalities are seeking help. They have only two things in common: heavy use of today's Internet porn and increasing need for more extreme material.[12]

But porn was available when we were kids, right? Wouldn't too much *Playboy* hurt sexual performance in the same way?

Not even close. The static images of *Playboy* can't compete with the readily available high-speed connection to the biggest database of porn in the world—the world wide web. Men are literally "numbing their brain's normal response to pleasure," and they can't "get it up" for their sexual partner anymore.[13]

That's scary! I don't want to fail in the bedroom because of an "affair" with virtual women on the screens in my house. Impotence is a natural consequence that I'd rather avoid. I think most teenagers would agree.

Porn has other natural consequences, like convincing our girls they are sex objects. Porn sites communicate two major lies to our young girls: You need to look perfect, and your value is based on sex. If our girls have frequented porn sites, we should engage in conversations about sexualization much as we discussed in chapter 6.

An important part of parenting is helping our kids recognize truth. Porn is a complete twisting of the truth. Real love takes work, patience, self-sacrifice, tenderness, and compassion. Real relationships are so much more than just sex. Porn, however, is just a sex show, where perfect-looking models engage in pure animalistic thrill with no concern for the long-term. Porn sets false expectations all around and eventually leads to disappointment with reality.

C. Establish Some Helpful Safeguards and Accountability

Again, a "Net Nanny" subscription might not be enough. Do you use parental controls on mobile devices? If you block porn on the router level, can your kids access your neighbor's router? Do you have HBO, Showtime, or Cinemax on your TV? Do you use passwords? Is your password your birthdate?

If you don't know exactly how to respond or what safeguards to implement, try asking your kid for their thoughts. Ask them, "What do you think would be good safeguards we can put in place to help you flee this temptation?" Read 1 Corinthians chapter 6 together and ask your kids, "Why does the apostle Paul use the word *flee* here?" And, "What do you think you could do to flee this type of temptation in the future?"

Remember, when your child turns eighteen, he or she is an adult and can do pretty much whatever they want. Try your best to help them build good habits and give them the tools to succeed on their own. Teach them to make good choices.

Porn can become a severe addiction. In some cases, children might need some professional help. Don't assume this right away, though. Don't make them feel like perverts. Don't overreact and start threatening to send them to a counselor. But if you think the problem is severe, don't hesitate to get a second opinion from a professional. Family counseling can be a very healthy thing.

Porn is a powerful enemy that seeks to destroy anyone it can get in its clutches. Young people and teenagers are particularly vulnerable to this monster. If your teenagers are among the unfortunate users of pornography, prepare yourself to be willing to make some big changes in your family's life for the sake of your kids.

Yes . . . this might mean canceling that HBO subscription.

Let's be honest. How well does the "Do what I say, not what I do" approach to parenting work? If we are watching inappropriate material ourselves, (1) our kids will most likely crack our codes and find it, (2) we are now opening the doors to material that objectifies women, and (3) we're being hypocritical bringing other people into our marital beds (yes, that's what lusting does).

Maybe we need to ask ourselves if *we* are fleeing sexual immorality.

Sexual immorality was a real struggle for many of the heroes in the Bible (Abraham, Judah, David, Solomon . . .) and it's a struggle for godly men and women today. Our kids aren't immune from it . . . and neither are we.

Are you being proactive or reactive about porn in your house?

10

Providing Answers About Masturbation

The answers to questions they're too embarrassed to ask

In Ron Howard's classic movie *Parenthood*, single parent Helen discovers a bunch of pornography in her son Garry's bedroom.

Unsure of how to respond, she asks her daughter's boyfriend, Tod, if he will talk to Garry. Tod is happy to oblige.

Later, after his conversation with Garry, Tod approaches Helen and tells her that Garry has been masturbating and felt like a pervert. Garry was very relieved when Tod told him, "That's what little dudes do."

That's what little dudes do.

Is that true?

Is masturbating just . . . *normal*?

Masturbating is a huge issue for young people. How huge? It's difficult to put numbers to it. Sure, plenty have taken surveys, but as a guy who looks at a lot of surveys and studies, I can tell you that these numbers vary a lot. I've seen surveys revealing that over

90 percent of males and females masturbate in any given year. Others show less than 50 percent for females.

One of the comprehensive studies I quoted earlier in the book, *The Social Organization of Sexuality*, surveyed people ages 18 to 59. Of those aged 18 to 24, 58 percent of men admitted to masturbation, and 41 percent of women. When the same age group was asked if they did it once a week, only 29 percent of men and 9 percent of women admitted to that frequency. That same survey asked the respondents how many felt guilty after masturbating. Fifty-four percent of men said they did, and 46 percent of women.[1]

But this survey was taken in 1992, before Internet porn was readily available. What about more recent studies?

Seventeen magazine currently reports that over 80 percent of guys masturbate, while only 60 percent of girls do.[2] *U.S. News* reported similar numbers from a National Survey of Sexual Health and Behavior in 2011. But this study was more specific about age:

> For both sexes, the likelihood of engaging in masturbation appeared to increase with age. Among boys between the ages of 14 and 17 the percentage of those who had masturbated at least once rose from about 63 to 80 percent. Among girls, those figures were lower but still followed an upward slope, rising from about 43 percent to 58 percent across the same time-frame, according to the report.[3]

Let me just say, I've met very few men (just two, actually, in my entire life) who told me they *didn't* masturbate regularly in their teen years. The percentages are very high for boys; I think it is easily 90 percent or more.

This isn't surprising. Males are more visual than females in a world overflowing with sexually charged images, and the male sex drive is strong . . . out of control, at times.

This doesn't mean females have no sex drive. Some are very driven by sex, and others experiment, curious about something so desired by most of the world.

Regardless of the exact numbers, it seems that over half of young people are doing it.

Plus, today's young people are waiting until their late twenties, on average, to get married, so must resist sexual temptation far longer. Fewer of today's twentysomethings are married than any generation prior at the same age. A 2014 PewResearch report revealed that only a quarter of Millennials are married. When previous generations were the age that Millennials are now, 36 percent of Generation X, 48 percent of baby boomers and 65 percent of the members of the Silent Generation were married.[4]

Grandma and Grandpa didn't have to wait as long for sex. And they didn't have to dodge porn on every screen either.

Let's just say masturbation seems like a solution for many. Not to mention that our world doesn't see any problem with it. Some doctors actually recommend it, calling it the "safest sex," healthy for your prostate (men), and a huge stress release.

Is the world right?

Is masturbation no big deal?

How should we respond if we suspect our kids are masturbating? Should we respond at all? If so, what do we communicate about this embarrassing subject?

Young Kids

First, understand that the word *masturbation* might insinuate many different acts. Toddlers might find that it feels good when they slide down the pole on the playground. I wouldn't call this masturbation.

My friend recently asked for advice. "My four-year-old likes rubbing her crotch against the car seat because it feels good. Sometimes she'll keep doing it throughout a car ride. Should I make her stop?"

I think the most important response is to avoid overreaction. No, your daughter isn't a pervert, and she isn't destined to be a stripper someday.

It might be time to open up some of those books about sexuality, body parts, and the changes we all go through, though. (I highlighted some of those in chapter 3.) During some of these casual and calm talks, a parent can mention how these parts are very special and will be used to make babies someday. If the "crotch grinding" continues, you could probably just casually ask her to stop doing it in the way you'd ask her to stop picking her nose.

I've talked with numerous parents who have dealt with this, and in most cases it was just a phase and it passed. Don't freak out.

Puberty

Once kids hit puberty, they might discover that it feels good when they touch their genitals, and they might experiment with it. This could start out as a pretty innocent act. Many young people might describe it as, "It tickles."

Again, this often can be an innocent exploration of the human body, and it contrasts greatly with the person who is viewing porn, lusting, and masturbating.

Does one lead to the other?

Again, when should a parent be worried? Should we even address this?

Looking for Answers

I remember the first time I discovered something "tingly" below the waist. I was about eleven years old. I hadn't gone through puberty (I was a late bloomer—all of my friends had body hair before I did), but I realized it felt good when I rubbed my penis a certain way in the sheets of my bed. Sometimes I found myself doing it until I reached orgasm.

I didn't do this every day, and I really don't recall thinking about girls or the female body when I did it. I just remember it feeling good.

By sixth grade my interest in the fairer sex had increased logarithmically. Sexual imagery began catching my eye, and I was distracted when my female classmates wore tight or revealing clothing.

One day in seventh grade, I distinctly remember overhearing a girl talking with her friends about watching a guy "jacking off." She made a hand gesture and I remember thinking, *How would that work?* That night I tried it . . . and I was hooked!

I can't tell you the exact moment, but masturbation quickly became a sexual thing for me. It wasn't just some innocent tingly feeling anymore. I thought about girls when I masturbated, and by twelve, as I shared in the previous chapter, I began viewing or thinking about pornographic images, and those always led me to masturbate.

The mind is a powerful thing.

At this point, the act of masturbation always made me feel guilty. I knew what lust was . . . *and I was definitely lusting.*

It became a habit, something I continued through much of my teen years. It's something I never brought up to anyone, something I was embarrassed by, but it was also something I really wanted deliverance from.

My dad subscribed me to a Christian magazine at the time, *Campus Life*. Each issue had a column about sex. Every time I received an issue I immediately turned to the sex column and read what the author had to say. He occasionally addressed issues like lust, but he rarely mentioned masturbation. I was always disappointed with what I read because the author never addressed the specific questions I had.

No one used the words I had heard.

No one addressed the thoughts I had.

No one was willing to talk about the truth in explicit detail.

Today's kids have numerous unanswered questions about this topic. I know, because every time I talk to young people about the subject, they approach me afterward to ask questions. And whenever we offer a question box for kids to ask anonymous questions, you'd be shocked to hear the kinds of questions they ask.

Our kids have questions; some of them have to do with masturbation.

Will they come to you for answers?

Getting Explicit

Near the beginning of this book I mentioned a study from the journal *Pediatrics* entitled, "Beyond the 'Big Talk,'" encouraging parents to consider having repeated discussions with their children about many aspects of sex instead of just one "big talk." The study concluded that "the more parents talked with their children, the closer their relationships." But I think the most fascinating aspect of this study was the benefit of speaking more explicitly.

Don't let the world *explicit* scare you. By explicit, I don't mean "naughty" or "inappropriate." I mean it in the true sense of the word. *Explicit* just means clear, overt, and unambiguous. Often, parents tend to be the opposite concerning the subject of sex. Parents are usually hesitant, vague, and ambiguous. In extreme examples, parents will avoid even saying certain words, or just say "down there" when referring to genitals or body parts. This subtly tells our kids that the subject is naughty and should be hush-hush.

I realize this can be embarrassing, but don't give in to the temptation to hush the subject. The *Pediatrics* study above revealed that the relationship between parent and child really "benefitted when the discussions moved beyond 'safe' or impersonal subjects such as puberty, reproduction and sexually transmitted diseases to more private topics such as masturbation and how sex feels."[5]

In other words, kids have explicit questions, and they appreciate it when their parents give them explicit answers.

Another study out of Montreal a few years ago revealed that more teens relied on advice from their parents than any other source. The advice of friends and celebrities ranked notably lower on the list than parents. Sadly, the same study revealed that 78 percent of moms believed their children looked chiefly to their friends for guidance on sexual behavior. In other words, parents ranked as the number one influence, but most of them thought their kids' friends were number one, so many parents sort of gave up even trying, ignorant of the impact they actually had.[6]

Don't give up. Your kids need to hear from you.

Are you ready to be a source of explicit truth about sex and even masturbation?

I find that today's young believers have two major questions about masturbation:

1. Is masturbation wrong?
2. If it is wrong, how can I stop?

Let's look at these answers explicitly.

Is Masturbation Wrong?

The Bible never uses the word *masturbation*. It talks about sex plenty, but the closest it comes to talking about masturbation is when a guy named Onan was supposed to provide an offspring for his brother's wife, and instead of doing his duty . . . well . . . Genesis 38 tells the story rather explicitly:

> So whenever he slept with his brother's wife, he spilled his semen on the ground to keep from providing offspring for his brother. What he did was wicked in the Lord's sight; so the Lord put him to death also.
>
> vv. 9–10 NIV

I guess I missed that *Veggie Tales* video.

This wasn't masturbation. This was the "withdrawal method" of birth control. (It's amazing how reading the Bible with your kids at the dinner table will springboard quite a few discussions about sex.)

The Bible doesn't address masturbation specifically, but it certainly addresses lust.

We've talked about God's plan for sex explicitly in chapter 4, so no need to rehash everything. But let's look at the highlights and then specifically at lust.

As we know, God's plan was made plain in the garden: A husband and a wife are to be united as one in the flesh. But some people didn't want to stick to their own spouses. They wanted others too, or they didn't want to wait for marriage. So God made it obvious, starting with the Ten Commandments in Exodus 20:14: "You must not commit adultery."

That's pretty clear. Don't have sex outside of marriage.

Then in the New Testament, the apostle Paul communicates on the topic in many passages, very explicitly in 1 Corinthians 6:18: "Run from sexual sin! No other sin so clearly affects the body as this one does. For sexual immorality is a sin against your own body."

Again, the term *sexual sin* means "the voluntary sex of an unmarried person." In other words, run from any temptation to have sex with someone you're not married to. Paul uses this term multiple times throughout his letters in the New Testament, usually saying something like flee from it, or have nothing to do with it.

But sadly, humans always try to come up with excuses for our sins. That's what the religious people did back in Jesus' day. They thought they could get away with *thinking* about sex as long as they didn't actually *do it*. Jesus himself decided to address this, calling it lust and labeling it just as bad as adultery.

> You have heard the commandment that says, "You must not commit adultery." But I say, anyone who even looks at a woman with lust has already committed adultery with her in his heart. So if your eye—even your good eye—causes you to lust, gouge it out and throw it away. It is better for you to lose one part of your body than for your whole body to be thrown into hell.
>
> Matthew 5:27–29

Jesus wasn't known for tiptoeing around issues. He was loving, he was merciful, he was forgiving . . . but when it came to religious people trying to justify their sins, he was forthright and frank. *Don't lust. You might as well have sex with someone who is not your wife, because it's the exact same thing. I look at the heart, not the fake actions you parade around!*

Paul chimes in on the same idea, advising us to flee "youthful lusts" (2 Timothy 2:22).

So we know that sex was created for marriage, sex outside of marriage is wrong, and if we think we are being good because we just imagine having sex with someone we aren't married to . . . we should pluck our eyes out!

So let me ask you. Is masturbating while looking at porn wrong?

The answer is pretty clear. Lusting is wrong. If we think we're not sinning when we look at or imagine pictures of people we're not married to, then we're fooling ourselves.

Let me say it again. Lusting is wrong. If we lust while masturbating, then it's wrong.

Now, I've met the occasional person who tells me, "I don't lust when I masturbate. It just feels good."

Here's my opinion about that:

If you're a guy, you're not only an adulterer, you're now also a liar. The male plumbing doesn't work that way. We don't achieve orgasm while thinking about Hannibal marching across the Alps with his elephants. I've talked with countless teenagers about masturbation in my twenty-plus years of youth ministry, listening to their candid confessions, and have never encountered a kid who thought about his geometry homework while masturbating. He might have been thinking about curves . . . but not the ones in geometry class.

Guys lust when they masturbate. End of story. Don't bring up the mentally insane or serial killers who actually masturbate to acts of violence. . . . Yes . . . these people do exist. But I don't think anyone wants to try to frame an argument that, "At least a serial killer isn't lusting while he kills someone."

Sure, if a married man masturbates while thinking of his wife, that's not sin. God knows our hearts and our minds. He knows exactly what we're thinking about. If we're lusting about someone other than our wife . . . it's sin.

I've also heard single guys argue, "I'm thinking about my future wife when I masturbate, so it's okay."

Again, I realize that this is a difficult temptation. But let's not distort truth to rationalize sin. I always reply to this argument by pointing out that if a guy is thinking about someone who is his "future wife" . . . she ain't his wife yet. If a cop caught him looking in her window, he couldn't argue, "But that's my wife!"

The officer of the law would ask, "Then why are you out here in the bushes looking in her window if that's your wife?"

"Well . . . it's my future wife."

Try that one sometime and see how far it gets you. (And God's a little smarter than most cops . . . no disrespect to my friends in blue.)

Most males, if we're being completely transparent, lust when we masturbate. And lusting after anyone but your spouse is adultery.

As for girls, I'll be bold enough to say that lust is usually the primary factor. Can I say without a doubt that is always the case? I'm a male, so I'll have to say the jury is still out on this one. Many females admit to thinking about erotic situations while they masturbate, but many also claim to be "just spacing out."

The female body works much different than the male. Males strive for a climax, and once they orgasm, they're done. Guys are all about the climax. Females can be more sensitive throughout the whole act. They might climax multiple times or not at all.

Some females argue that women who masturbate are just filling a void or have attachment issues. Others in the Christian community have spoken out against these claims, like Jordon Monge in her *Christianity Today* article, "The Real Problem with Female Masturbation." The subtitle of the article is "Call it what it is: Ladies who lust."

Monge contends:

> We need a strategy that recognizes the sin of lust and calls it by its name, rather than pretending that women have no agency beyond reacting to environmental stressors or psychological difficulties. We must treat lust like other sins—not a way we act out as a consequence of other problems in our lives—but as a sin requiring us to learn the discipline of self-control that we must master if we ever hope to be the women God made us to be.[7]

I'm not going to point any fingers, because I can't tell a female how she feels. But I can say this: If we are lusting, we need to call it what it is. More important, we need to look for ways to help our kids flee these temptations.

Helping Our Kids Break Free

The best way to help our kids break free of masturbation is to be *proactive* about it instead of *reactive*. Too often, we wait until something is a problem before we address it, when it's a topic we should have been addressing all along. We have to be proactively teaching about lust in the context of our continual conversations about sex.

Yes, I'm repeating something I've said in the previous nine chapters, and I'll probably repeat it again in the next two. It's the theme of this whole book: *Don't be afraid to engage in frequent conversations sharing the explicit truth about sex.*

I know when I was a teenager struggling with lust and masturbation, I was looking for answers. I had heard plenty of people say, "Wait until marriage for sex." And frankly, I bought that (not all teenagers do). But not many people in my life were talking about the particulars like lust, pornography, masturbation, and how far was just far enough.

We need to constantly communicate the truth about what God thinks about lust.

You might remember a surprising fact I shared in chapter 4. The number one reason young people wait for sex is . . . *God.*

The Centers for Disease Control's National Survey of Family Growth report revealed the number one reason teenagers provided for waiting for sex was that it was "against religion or morals."[8] They waited because they knew it was the right thing to do.

How are our kids going to know the truth if we don't tell them? I guarantee they are hearing plenty of lies.

So engage in frequent conversations with your kids about porn, lust, and even the embarrassing topic of masturbation.

But don't just say, "Don't do it." Tell your kids how. Give your kids some tools and ammo to flee those temptations.

First, provide the knowledge of the importance of fleeing. Take a passage we've discussed before and talk about it, like the 2 Timothy 2:22 verse about fleeing youthful lusts:

> Run from anything that stimulates youthful lusts. Instead, pursue righteous living, faithfulness, love, and peace. Enjoy the companionship of those who call on the Lord with pure hearts.

Ask your kids:

- What does this passage advise us to do with things in our life that might stimulate lust?
- Why do you think Paul tells us to run or flee from these?
- What are some of the things that might stimulate lusts in young people today?
- What are some of the temptations like this you face?
- How could you "run" from these?

I like using Scripture to combat the lies of this world. Let's be honest. Most young people aren't "fleeing" lust or sexual sin. Their playlists are full of sexually charged lyrics, and the images they watch on screens are full of racy visuals and "do what feels right at the moment" messages.

What do you think "feels right" when they encounter sexual temptations in the moment?

The key to fighting sexual sin is teaching our kids the power God gives us through a relationship with him and his Spirit living inside of us. The world loves to tell us to do whatever *we desire.* God's Word tells us to *let his Spirit guide us*.

> So I say, let the Holy Spirit guide your lives. Then you won't be doing what your sinful nature craves. The sinful nature wants to do evil, which is just the opposite of what the Spirit wants. And the Spirit gives us desires that are the opposite of what the sinful nature desires.
>
> Galatians 5:16–17

Are we teaching our kids to listen to God or to their own desires?

The age-old phrase "An ounce of prevention is worth a pound of cure" holds true with teaching our kids the truth about sex. The more we teach them about God's amazing creation and his love for us, the more they'll understand God's gift of sex, and the more they'll recognize any imitations.

John Piper provides some pretty good advice about battling lust in a very memorable acronym, ANTHEM.[9] His suggestions include avoiding temptation, saying no to lustful thoughts, and turning our minds toward Christ. Google "John Piper, ANTHEM" for the full explanation.

What can you do today to *not overreact*, but start calmly and casually *interacting* with your kids about God's amazing creation and his beautiful gift of sex?

11

Surviving a Blotted Past

Finding healing even if it feels too late

"It's too late."

I've heard it from teenagers countless times. They hear the truth about staying sexually pure until marriage, and they might even agree it sounds nice, but they've already engaged in some sort of sexual activity, and they feel *dirty,* or . . . *blemished*.

"I'm already *not* a virgin, so it doesn't matter now."

Past mistakes can leave a trail of hurt. A teen pregnancy, the inherent shame of being caught using pornography . . . Do these past experiences have to leave scars?

Sometimes hurt is inflicted on our kids in the form of sexual violation or abuse. Now they are feeling pain and regret for something that isn't even their fault. How can parents help their kids overcome this kind of hurt?

Keys for Parents

In this chapter we'll look at three steps to helping our kids overcome a blotted past. But first, let me share two very important reminders about our approach.

1. Don't Freak Out

Yeah, I've said it before in this book, and it's worth repeating. When Mom or Dad overreacts, it only widens the chasm between parent and child. I know, because when I've lost my temper with my own kids, the wounding results are undeniable.

Mental note: Don't be honest or vulnerable with Dad; he'll flip out!

If our kids are already experiencing hurt or guilt, the last thing they need is to have to manage an emotionally unstable parent.

I have a friend who got pregnant as a teen. Her parents kicked her out of the house immediately and she had to fend for herself. She not only felt guilty for her mistake, she felt abandoned and alone.

I have another good friend who was abused by her brother when she was a child. Her mother went into a rage—demanding to know all the details, asking her where she was touched, dragging her to the doctor, and making a huge scene. Every time her mom brought it up, which was way too often, she would turn away from her daughter with a look of disgust. My friend was only eight at the time. She was left feeling dirty and ashamed.

Years later that friend of mine went to counseling. Her psychologist told her that her mother's reaction was probably equally, if not more, harmful than the original abuse.

Our reactions matter.

When our kids experience hurt, self-inflicted or not, they need someone safe.

Are you that person?

I wonder that myself. Will my daughter come to me with her pain and tough questions?

If you discover your kid's imperfect past, don't blow a gasket. Take time if you need it and figure out how you can transform your overreaction into interaction. Don't let your emotions inhibit the opportunity to walk through this experience with your child, providing love, grace, and healing.

Chances are you have some blotches on your record too. Approach your kids with the compassion of a fellow sinner. Jesus has offered us a fresh start.

And that leads me to my second reminder.

2. Don't Dwell on the Past

As parents, we can help our kids see the freedom from a blotted past that Jesus provides.

Past imperfections shouldn't impede fresh futures . . . especially when Jesus offers us a new beginning. Think about that. *A new beginning*. I don't know many teenagers who wouldn't want a "do-over."

Do your teenagers know they can have a do-over?

If you read the Gospels, you'll notice that imperfect people seemed especially attracted to Jesus. In fact, the more messed up they were, the more they wanted to meet this guy, who offered repentance and a fresh start.

Sadly, Christians don't always reflect Jesus. Christians can be pretty condemning at times. If they'd open their Bibles and read about Jesus, they'd discover he didn't come to condemn. Point of fact, the verse immediately after the most popular verse in the Bible says just that: "God did not send his Son into the world to condemn the world, but to save the world through him" (John 3:17 NIV).

Jesus didn't focus on blemished pasts; he focused on a fresh future. That means even if our kids have already been sexually active, frequented porn sites, or become slaves to masturbation . . . it's not too late.

Parents can help their kids find healing when it feels too late.

Not My Kid

Here's where most parents might be tempted to say, "Well, luckily my kid hasn't done any of that."

It would be rather optimistic of me to assume every parent who reads this book is going to sit down and have conversations with their eight-, ten-, or twelve-year-old, just in time to help them make good decisions about sex before they've gone down a different path.

But what if your kids are older? We don't want to assume the worst, but what if they've already experimented sexually like so many teens do? Looking back at the numbers shared earlier in this book, one-third of U.S. high school freshmen and almost two-thirds of high school seniors have already had sexual intercourse.[1] And the previous two chapters revealed an overwhelming majority of kids who have viewed pornography or struggle with masturbation. Statistically, many of our teenagers have already made some of these decisions.

Sadly, some of our kids didn't even make decisions, but had decisions made for them. Later in this chapter we'll see that anywhere from one in five to a shocking one in three youth have been sexually abused or victimized. How can we help them overcome that kind of pain?

Our kids might feel that some of these past experiences will taint them for life.

How can we help them survive the past and look forward to a bright future?

Let's first look at what we can do to help our kids who have already been sexually active, frequented porn sites, or struggle with masturbation. Then let's look at what we can do if our kids have been sexually abused or victimized.

Helping Kids Overcome a Blotted Past

If our teenagers have already struggled with lust or masturbation or engaged in sexual activity, they aren't dirty or blemished. They're human. They're sinners like the rest of us, and we all desperately need Jesus. I know I do.

Jesus has offered us a fresh start. As parents, we can help our kids see the freedom Jesus provides from a blotted past.

Here are three steps that can help our kids overcome past imperfections and look forward to a bright future.

1. Accept Forgiveness for the Past

Guilt is a cumbersome burden. Some choose to drag it around for life. This is even more common with sexual mistakes. Promiscuous activity has always been hushed in the church. So if our kids mess up in this area, why would they want to bring it to light? The natural tendency is to bury it and hope it goes away.

Sadly, burying sin never works. It tends to rot and grow into something bigger. That's probably why the Bible encourages us to confess our sins to one another (James 5:16). Not as some religious ritual that we have to do . . . but because we want freedom from the bondage that sin brings.

We can help our kids find freedom from the chains of guilt by pointing them to the fresh start Jesus provides. The more we spend time reading the Bible, the more we'll see examples of this.

Look at the story of Jonah and Nineveh. An entire city was evil and corrupt, but God chose to have compassion on them. Funny, God's compassion was so great it made Jonah mad. Jonah was actually hoping God would destroy the city.

This is a good life lesson for our kids. Sometimes God's people aren't as forgiving as God is. God is willing to forget our sins and free us from our blotted past.

The New Testament provides countless examples of this as well: the story of the woman at the well in John chapter 4, the story of Zachaeus in Luke chapter 19 . . . Jesus didn't hold their pasts against them. Instead, he offered them forgiveness and a bright future.

One of the best examples of this is in John chapter 8, where the Pharisees bring a woman caught in the act of adultery to Jesus, demanding he tell them what to do with her.

This had to be mortifying for the woman. Sure, she had messed up, but these religious snobs were using her to try to trap Jesus. Jesus was in a Catch-22. If he said, "Stone her," then the Pharisees would go to the Romans and get Jesus busted for carrying out capital punishment without permission. On the other hand, if he said, "Let her go," they would blame him for not following the Old Testament civil law punishing adulterers.

In the midst of this trap, Jesus shows compassion for the woman.

> They were trying to trap him into saying something they could use against him, but Jesus stooped down and wrote in the dust with his finger. They kept demanding an answer, so he stood up again and said, "All right, but let the one who has never sinned throw the first stone!" Then he stooped down again and wrote in the dust.
>
> When the accusers heard this, they slipped away one by one,

> beginning with the oldest, until only Jesus was left in the middle of the crowd with the woman. Then Jesus stood up again and said to the woman, "Where are your accusers? Didn't even one of them condemn you?"
>
> "No, Lord," she said.
>
> And Jesus said, "Neither do I. Go and sin no more."
>
> John 8:6–11

This is one of those Bible passages where everyone tries to speculate about something *not* in the text. We don't know what Jesus was writing in the ground.

Guess what?

It doesn't matter.

Here's what matters: When this woman is dragged in front of the crowd either naked or wrapped in a sheet . . . *all eyes are on her*. This woman has probably never felt the fear and shame that she is feeling at this moment.

So what does Jesus do?

He starts doodling in the sand.

Where is everyone's attention now?

Jesus takes the attention off of her and *onto his doodling*. Better yet, he repels her accusers. Jesus brings up the sin of each of these hypocrites and basically tells them, "Sure, if you guys have never sinned, then go ahead and start throwing rocks!"

They all go away, defeated in this particular battle of wits. Why? Because none of them can deny that they are sinners.

That's a good lesson for us, as parents, to remember if our kids make mistakes like these. We're all sinners. We all make mistakes. And Jesus offers us a fresh start if we're willing to accept his forgiveness.

First John 1:8–9 spells it out:

> If we claim we have no sin, we are only fooling ourselves and not living in the truth. But if we confess our sins to him, he is faithful and just to forgive us our sins and to cleanse us from all wickedness.

Jesus offers us a fresh start. He is willing to cleanse us from our past mistakes.

The more we share the stories of Jesus with our kids, the more they'll see that he doesn't care about the mistakes of our past, he cares about our future.

Jesus' words are powerful in the ending to that story above. He asks the woman if anyone stuck around to condemn her. There's that word *condemn* again. It seems like church people often think we are supposed to condemn sinners, but they will never find Scripture to back it up. Jesus didn't come to condemn, and he didn't let it happen to this adulterer. No one stuck around to condemn her because they all knew they were imperfect just like her.

That's why he said, "Neither do I. Go and sin no more."

There's that same theme again: *I don't condemn you for your past, but I care about your future.*

Which leads us to the second step we can teach our kids.

2. Don't Let Past Missteps Justify Future Mistakes

God's grace isn't a license to sin even more.

Sometimes when we hear about how compassionate and forgiving God is, we use that as an excuse to sin even more. *After all, I can just ask for forgiveness later.*

This can hurt us two ways.

First and foremost, it hurts our relationship with God. The foundation of our relationship with God is based on our trust in him. How much are we trusting in him if we aren't willing to give everything to him?

Paul tackles this faulty logic in Romans chapter 6. He asks:

> Well then, should we keep on sinning so that God can show us more and more of his wonderful grace? Of course not! Since we have died to sin, how can we continue to live in it?
>
> Romans 6:1–2

Paul goes on to urge us to put our complete trust in God, warning, "Do not let sin control the way you live; do not give in to sinful desires" (v. 12).

Second, using past missteps as an excuse to justify future mistakes can also bring some pretty severe consequences. God is willing to forgive us, but that doesn't necessarily free us from natural consequences.

If your son gets his girlfriend pregnant, God's forgiveness doesn't free him from the ramifications of that decision.

If your daughter gets chlamydia and never realizes she has it (which happens frequently because the disease is asymptomatic), the consequences are often sterility.

Our choices have consequences. God's grace isn't a "get out of jail free" card for natural consequences.

My friend "Donna" learned that the hard way.

Donna was sexually active all through high school. She loved partying and having sex with anyone she wanted, and she got away with it for a while. But eventually her life of partying left her homeless and alone.

One day a couple from a local church met her on the street and offered her food to eat and eventually a place to stay. Donna thought, *Sure, I'll take advantage of these stupid people and rip them off when they sleep.* But each night when Donna went to bed she told herself, "I'll rip them off tomorrow." After all, the people were nice, the bed was comfortable, and she hadn't had good food like this in a long time.

As months passed, she became friends with the woman who had taken her in. Eventually Donna gave her life to Jesus, and he began to transform her.

One night Donna was in her old neighborhood and she encountered some friends she used to party with. They invited her to a party and Donna wondered what one party could hurt.

That night Donna made a decision that had some painful ramifications.

That night Donna got HIV.

God has forgiven Donna for every one of her mistakes, but Donna is still carrying the consequences in her numbered years.

Just because God offers us a clean slate, it doesn't give us license to do whatever we want.

That's probably why we should . . .

3. Make a Plan for the Future

The best thing we can do with past mistakes is *learn* from them.

When your kids mess up, help them make a plan to avoid the same mistake in the future. Use the same method we've discussed repeatedly in this book—engage in dialogue, not monologue.

When your kids mess up, don't automatically shift into lecture mode. I've made this mistake countless times with my kids. Kids don't need our lecturing. They need our listening.

So turn "You should . . ." into "What do you think you should you do?"

If your son got alone with a girl and found that "it was impossible to stop," don't lecture him. Instead, ask him, "What do you think you could do to avoid the situation in the future?"

This doesn't mean you don't share truth. Share, then ask questions. Tell him, "Most bad choices began five choices ago." Then ask him:

- What does that mean?
- What did that look like in this situation?
- How can you avoid this temptation in the future?
- What kind of conversation should you have with (girl's name)?

Share with him what the Bible says about fleeing. Ask him questions about what fleeing looks like in his world.

Past mistakes can be costly, but they can also be a great teaching tool, motivating us to make better choices for the future.

I also like to encourage kids to find someone they can talk with about sexual temptation. This creates accountability. Ask your child, "Who is someone you can call when you're feeling tempted? Who is someone who is putting God first in their own life who would encourage you to do the same?"

The Bible constantly encourages us to enlist others in this journey:

> Two people are better off than one, for they can help each other succeed. If one person falls, the other can reach out and help. But someone who falls alone is in real trouble.
>
> Ecclesiastes 4:9–10

Encourage your kids not to go on this journey alone.

Overcoming Sexual Abuse or Victimization

What if our kids have been sexually abused or victimized? What kind of help can we offer them?

First, realize they aren't alone.

Studies by David Finkelhor, Director of the Crimes Against Children Research Center, reveal:

- One in five girls and one in twenty boys is a victim of child sexual abuse.
- Twenty-eight percent of U.S. youth ages fourteen to seventeen said they had been sexually victimized at some time in their lives
- Children are most vulnerable to sexual abuse between the ages of seven and thirteen.[2]

According to a 2003 National Institute of Justice report, three out of four adolescents who have been sexually assaulted were victimized by someone they knew well.[3]

Young people carrying the burden of sexual abuse often feel dirty or used. Sadly, they might even feel it is their own fault. In most cases, professional help is recommended. But as parents, we too should be an encouragement to them about a bright future.

If your child has experienced sexual abuse, I recommend three steps.

Report It

Sometimes people avoid reporting abuse because of the pain and embarrassment, but this often leaves a predator free to do more harm. Most sexual predators act repeatedly. Your reporting could prevent countless future victims from the abuse or victimization your own child has endured. If you discover abuse or victimization, report it.

Seek Professional Help

This isn't something kids should be embarrassed about. Counselors can provide the tools individuals need to overcome past hurt. They can also provide parents some guidance on how to help kids heal.

Focus on the Future

Abuse victims often blame themselves and dwell on the past. As parents, we can not only assure them, "It's not your fault," but we can also help them look forward to a bright future. Introduce them to God's grace in every situation and show biblical examples of Jesus helping people overcome all kinds of pasts (like the previous examples in this chapter).

This kind of hurt is never easy. There is no magic Band-Aid that makes it all better after one application. This takes time, it takes care, and often takes professional help.

But Jesus offers a fresh start for everyone.

Everyone.

Recalculating

Have you ever veered off the path while on a road trip?

Ever take a wrong turn?

There is one word a GPS uses that we all know too well: "*Recalculating.*"

I might be driving to Los Angeles, but when I turn off the freeway to grab a Wendy's Frosty, a soft female voice calmly says, "Recalculating."

If road construction sends you miles off course and you have no idea where you are, the word *recalculating* actually brings hope. It's a voice that says, "I haven't given up. Sure, we've veered from our intended course, but I'm still going to get you there. Let's start again from this new location."

It would be pretty discouraging if our GPS said, "Pull over and shut off the ignition; you have passed the point of no return. This is where you are going to die."

My GPS has never done that. Instead . . . "Recalculating."

In other words, "Don't give up. We'll get there."

We can be that calm voice in our child's ear: "It's not too late. Jesus has offered us a fresh start."

Parents can help their kids find healing when it feels too late.

Jesus doesn't care about our past, he cares about our future. Walk with your kids on this journey and experience the freedom God provides.

12

Tough Questions

Answering difficult questions about sex and intimacy

"Is it okay if I masturbate to keep from looking at porn?"

"Is it wrong if I am attracted to someone of the same sex?"

"I just want to be loved, and the only way guys want me is if I give them sex. Does God want me to be alone?"

These are the kinds of questions asked by many young people today . . . and these questions, and more, are exactly what we're going to answer in this chapter.

Celebrate Questions

We can engage in countless conversations with our kids and they'll *still* come up and ask us tough questions. Sometimes these are questions we might feel like we've covered time and time again. But don't let this distress you.

Questions are good.

Questions mean you are a safe person to ask.

Questions mean you have created a comfortable climate where conversation is welcomed.

So don't be concerned when your kids ask you, "Is oral sex wrong?" The fact is, *they are asking you!* Celebrate the question.

In this chapter, I'll include the most common questions I've heard from young people in the last decade, and I'll also include many of the questions submitted by my blog readers at JonathanMcKeeWrites.com. I appealed to them, "Gimme the most common sex questions young people ask today," and they sent me a copious amount of current questions.

But before we dig in, let's remember a few principles that will help us keep these communication channels open:

1. Don't Freak Out:

Yes, I've already said it countless times in this book. But one last reminder doesn't hurt. Take a deep breath and thank God that your kids are asking you this question. Our calm responses will keep them coming to us.

2. Tell Me More:

If you are shocked by what they ask or you don't know the answer . . . stall! Say, "Tell me more about the context of this question so I can better answer it." Or feel free to just pause and say, "Great question. Hmmmmm. Let me think about that one for a moment." If you need more time to think about it or research it, tell them that. Or one better . . .

3. What do you think?

Let's face it, we aren't always going to be there. Someday they'll be in a college dorm, an army barracks, a nightclub (hopefully not, but possible), and they are going to have to ask themselves, "What is right?" Delight at every chance you get to help them practice problem solving and decision making. Ask them what they think.

Ask them what the Bible says about it. Get them used to learning how to discover answers.

So be prepared when your eighth-grade boy asks you, "If God only wants marriage to be for one man and one woman, how come almost every Bible hero has several wives?" Don't freak out. Tell him, "Great question." And if you need some time to think about the answer, ask him, "What do you think?"

Let's dig in.

Questions We've Already Answered

I'll start with some of the common questions that we've already touched on in this book. I'll answer them briefly, since they've been answered in detail elsewhere, then I'll tell you where you can read and review the answer.

Why should I wait until marriage to have sex? All my friends are doing it.

This is the most common question young people ask today. That's why we dedicated an entire chapter to this question—chapter 4. In fact, we answered this question biblically, scientifically, and logically.

I've already had sex; why bother to save myself anymore?

This is such a common question among young people. Sadly, many young people have a past and they think, *I'm already damaged goods.*

We covered the answer to this question extensively in chapter 11. No sin has dirtied us beyond redemption. Jesus offers us freedom from our past, and he wants us to trust him with our future. Past missteps don't justify future mistakes.

Is masturbation wrong?

We covered this question in detail in chapter 10. It's wrong when we lust, and most masturbation involves lust.

What counts as "sex," anyway?

We answered this question pretty clearly in chapters 4 and 5. Sex isn't just intercourse, it's an intimate process that begins when people "initiate the launch sequence." Anyone who has ever been in a moment of passion, even with all their clothes on, would attest to the intensity and heat of the moment. It's difficult to stop, simply because it's a process that's not supposed to be stopped. Anyone in that situation is clearly thinking sexual thoughts, and those moments are supposed to be reserved for marriage. When sexual thoughts are outside of marriage, they are lust.

So call me crazy when I label it *sexual immorality* when two teenagers lie down on a couch with their clothes on and make out passionately. Some thought Jesus was crazy when he told them, "But I say, anyone who even looks at a woman with lust has already committed adultery with her in his heart" (Matthew 5:28).

So what counts as sex? Any intimate physical activity that starts the engines roaring. These moments are meant for marriage, and they're amazing!

How far can I go?

This is very similar to the previous question. And we dedicated all of chapter 5 to answering it. The answer is, *As far as you'd go in front of your grandmother.*

What about abuse/rape?

We covered this common question in chapter 11. Jesus can heal us from past hurt and give us a fresh start.

This kind of hurt is never easy. There is no magic Band-Aid that makes it all better after one application. Healing takes time. So when you feel hopeless or ashamed, remember the three steps in chapter 11: report it, seek help, and focus on the future.

And don't forget to ask God for his help. Pray and specifically ask him for deliverance from feelings of guilt and shame. God can carry you through these tough times. Some of us don't reach out to him until we need him, but that doesn't stop him from being there.

Corrie ten Boom, a wise woman imprisoned for helping Jews escape the Nazi Holocaust, said, "You may never know that Jesus is all you need, until Jesus is all you have."

Jesus offers a fresh start for everyone.

Everyone.

New Questions

Here are some more questions young people commonly ask, along with some biblical answers.

Is it okay to send each other sexy pictures on our phones?

My guess is our kids already know the answer to this question.

Sure, the Bible *doesn't* say, "Thou shalt not sendeth naked pictures." True. But let's break this down from what we know the Bible *does* say.

If a girl sends her boyfriend a sexy picture, he is going to be tempted to lust, and lust is sin. We are supposed to flee this kind of temptation.

If a guy sends a girl a sexy picture, first, he's confused—most girls aren't visual like this. But second, if a girl is actually turned on by this, then she's lusting, and she shouldn't be doing it.

Sadly, a recent study showed that over half of teenagers have received or sent either sexually suggestive texts or pictures.[1] Similar studies show those teens are four to six times more likely to have sex than those teens who don't.[2] Think about it. If young people are thinking about sex and flirting with their girlfriend or boyfriend with sexually explicit messages, those actions eventually progress to something more—the complete opposite of fleeing sexual temptation.

So no, our kids shouldn't send sexy pictures until they're married. And even then, I would warn them to be careful sending sexy pictures to their spouse because for whatever reason, those pictures have the potential of getting out. That kind of fun should be saved for the bedroom, where there's no chance of pictures showing up on the Internet someday and ruining their life.

Can I have sex when I'm engaged?

This is another great question, and it's usually asked by someone who doesn't necessarily want to know the truth as much as they want to find some justification for their actions. How do I know this? Because not only have I addressed this question from young men countless times . . . *I asked this question myself when I was engaged!* (And I only wanted to hear one answer.)

Sometimes young people will even arm themselves with verses to support their claim. And in today's world, they can Google it and find someone who argues premarital sex for engaged couples. The logic usually sounds something like this:

> In Bible times, the betrothal period was very much like our engagement, and as we know from Deuteronomy 20:7, it's okay to sleep with our fiancé during this period. We've both been pure so far, so now that we've found that special someone and have committed to each other in this engagement, isn't it okay to go ahead and share that intimate bond? After all, it's for two people who want to spend the rest of their lives together, right? And we are exactly that! Who says we need to wait for a piece of paper when it's really God who joins us together?

Yeah . . . I've heard all of that, including the very poor interpretation of Deuteronomy 20:7.

First, let's be clear. God's plan for marriage is unmistakable in the Bible. Reread chapter 4 of this book. It's all laid out. Husband and wife. Not fiancés.

Second, the betrothal period was way more serious than an engagement. It's hardly a comparison. It was a very serious commitment, so much so that you actually had to divorce to get out of it. You might recall the example of Mary and Joseph. Joseph was "pledged to be married" to Mary (Matthew 1:18 NIV), but then she got pregnant: "Because Joseph her husband was faithful to the law, and yet did not want to expose her to public disgrace, he had in mind to divorce her quietly" (Matthew 1:19 NIV).

This "divorce" was from the betrothal. Serious stuff.

Third, it wasn't God's plan for betrothed couples to have sex. People might try to cite verses like Deuteronomy 20:7 that seem like exceptions, but look up that verse for yourself. Depending on the version you have, it will read something like this:

> Has anyone here just become engaged to a woman but not yet married her? Well, you may go home and get married! You might die in the battle and someone else would marry her.
>
> Deuteronomy 20:7

Some think that this can be interpreted as "go home and sleep with her."

It's funny how people love to try to find one exception from an Old Testament civil or ceremonial law and use it as the justification for their actions rather than seeking what God's Word says repeatedly throughout Scripture: *No sex outside of marriage, either adultery or sexual immorality*. In chapter 4 of this book we looked at numerous verses sharing this truth, including Hebrews 13:4, addressing both adultery and fornication: "Marriage should be honored by all, and the marriage bed kept pure, for God will judge the adulterer and all the sexually immoral" (NIV).

Fourth (yeah, I even have a fourth reason), I've met countless couples who were engaged only to break up before the wedding. This just happened to a close friend of ours. What then?

Sex is reserved for marriage. Not engagement, not some exception of betrothal . . . *just marriage*.

So if you want to have sex with your fiancé, then get married.

Is it wrong to lie in a bed, but not have sex, with your significant other?

Let's be honest. Men have a huge sex drive, and I don't know a single man who wouldn't be tempted lying in bed with a female.

The Bible repeatedly says, "Flee sexual immorality." Lying in a bed together is the complete opposite of fleeing. This would tempt any man with a pulse.

Why would God, who says that all he created was good, tell us that we can't have sex whenever we want?

This is a great question, and it's really a matter of perspective.

When young people ask this question, they are living in a small time period of their lives where sexual temptation is very difficult and very real. For my great grandpa, this was only a few years. Kids were beginning puberty later, and they were getting married earlier. He was married at eighteen. He probably only endured a few years of sexual temptation.

I began puberty a little earlier and got married at twenty, so I was tempted sexually for almost eight years.

My son went through puberty earlier than I did and he's now twenty-one as I write this, and he's not close to getting married. For young people today these years might seem long and arduous. So from their perspective, they might see it as torture and question why God would make them endure such suffering.

A few thoughts I share with young people:

1. Don't wait so long for marriage.

In 1 Corinthians 7:9 Paul writes, "But if they cannot control themselves, they should marry, for it is better to marry than to burn with passion" (NIV). Today's young people seem to want to finish college and grad school and pay off loans before getting married. And one reason they aren't in a hurry to marry is because they're sleeping around anyway. That's not God's plan. If two people really want to get married, they can make it happen. It might take sacrifice, but it's possible. I know. My wife and I were twenty and twenty-one years old when we got married.

2. Don't date until you're ready.

You don't need an exclusive boyfriend or girlfriend when you're twelve years old. I know, it's hard, because every Disney channel show you watched growing up shows sixth graders pursuing dating relationships, and your friends are all pursuing them too. Dating isn't bad, but ask yourself, "Where's the future in this?" Date when you're good and ready to find a suitable companion. Until then, enjoy plenty of friends of the opposite sex.

3. Waiting for sex is a discipline and well worth the price.

Genesis tells us the story of a man named Jacob who was so in love with the woman he wanted to marry that he worked seven years to marry her. (Then ended up working seven more). Ask your teens, "How hard are you willing to work for the man/woman you love? How much are you willing to endure?" These years might be tough, but discipline yourself to simply enjoy the friendship of the opposite sex until you get married, even those whom you date. Don't give in to the pressure that dating equals getting hot and heavy. Enjoy companionship and great conversation now, then enjoy a lifetime of great sex. The alternative is to enjoy a promiscuous lifestyle for a few years right now and then suffer the consequences of that promiscuity for a lifetime. Your choice.

Is premarital oral sex wrong?

When I'm asked questions like this, I like to answer with a question. "What do you think?"

My kids have asked me this question, and that's exactly how I responded. I asked them their opinion. They thought it was fine for marriage; after all, the Bible never addresses it as a sin. It's just another intimate sexual act between a husband and a wife. I told them, "I agree."

But when our kids ask if oral sex is okay outside of marriage, I'd ask them, "What does the Bible tell us about sexual acts outside of marriage?" This goes back to what we discussed in detail in chapters 4 and 5. For those who would argue it's not sex, I would refer to Jesus' teaching that lust is adultery. And I don't know many people who can have oral sex without having sexual thoughts. It's an intimate sexual act, and intimate sexual acts are reserved for marriage.

If a guy has anal sex with a girl, are they still virgins?

Anal sex is a sexual act. If a couple engages in anal sex instead of intercourse so they can stay sexually pure, they're fooling themselves. Just like oral sex, anal sex is a type of sexual activity where you are undoubtedly having sexual thoughts. If you do this outside of marriage, then it's sexual immorality, which is sin.

In addition, people who have anal sex can experience some potential unwanted effects like hemorrhoids or even tearing. It's not a popular subject to talk about, but the fact is, God made the vagina self-lubricating and perfect for the act of making love. When couples try anal sex, they usually use a lubricant, and they have to wash really well when finished. Even then, the woman might get hemorrhoids or experience tearing. Most doctors would recommend extreme caution.

Is it okay if I masturbate to keep from looking at porn?

I'd answer this question with a question: "Is masturbation wrong?" (We answered this one clearly in chapter 10. It's wrong when you lust, which is most masturbation.)

Then I'd ask, "Is it okay to do one sin to keep from doing another?"

Sin has consequences, period. Help your kids seek out other ways to flee porn rather than masturbating while lusting in their minds. (Flip back to the previous chapters and look at some of those suggestions once again for fleeing pornography and other sexual temptations.)

Is it good to masturbate before a date to "flee" having sex with my girlfriend?

This is almost the same question as above, but with a little added use of Scripture. Just as Satan twisted Scripture to tempt Jesus, sometimes people will twist Scripture to try to justify sins.

No, same as above. One sin doesn't justify another. If you want to "flee" having sex with your girlfriend, avoid tempting situations. Go to dinner and then hang out with some friends. Don't get alone with her.

If marriage is for one man and one woman, how come so many Bible heroes had multiple wives?

God's plan was laid out clearly in the garden. One man, one woman, to become one in the flesh. That plan never changed. But people strayed from God's plan regardless.

The Old Testament stories often tell us all the explicit details, but within those details lies the explicit truth.

For example: Abraham didn't trust God's promise for a son, so he slept with Hagar. Seem like no big deal? This single decision caused fighting, jealousy, and chaos that has lasted for thousands of years.

Jacob was tricked into his first marriage, so he married again. When those two wives didn't produce like Jacob wanted, he slept with two other women. These decisions caused competition, quarreling, and jealousy for generations to come.

God instructed his kings to be an example to God's people and only take one wife (Deuteronomy 17:14–20). Most of them didn't abide, and the result was consequences of the worst kind.

God's plan for one husband and one wife is clearly the best plan.

If you really investigate the Scripture, it's plainly evident that God's way is so much better than our way. The Old Testament stories demonstrate that.

At the same time, these stories demonstrate that God can use sinful people, blemishes and all. Yes, these people would have avoided many natural consequences had they listened to God in the first place. But God uses us despite our mistakes.

I just want to be loved, and the only way guys want me is if I give them sex. Does God want me to be alone?

In chapter 8, I made a statement:

Guys give love to get sex.

Girls give sex to get love.

No, not all guys are evil manipulators, and no, not all girls are seductive temptresses. But sadly, many young men and women drift toward each of these roles today.

Guys are so driven by their libidos they will often do almost anything to fulfill them. Girls are often so desperate to find a guy who actually cares, they will sacrifice their own moral code to get one.

I like to ask my daughters, "What characteristics are you looking for in a husband?"

As they describe a perfect man, my guess is, they are *not* going to describe the kind of guy who only wants a girl if she gives him sex.

We need to affirm that our daughters are valuable, and encourage them not to lower their standards just because it seems like the "pickings are slim." Frankly, the pickings are often slim because our daughters are looking in the wrong places.

Where do girls look for guys today? If they believe current popular songs, then they'll put on a tight dress, "drink it up," and "drop it low" at a nightclub. If they believe Scripture, then they're going to "devote themselves to fellowship" among other things (Acts 2:42), and meet others who are devoted to Christ.

I tell my girls that if they want to meet a godly man, hang out where godly men are. My girls are both involved in ministry at their church, go on annual mission trips, and know numerous godly young men.

If a guy demands sex from a girl, he's not a guy worth having.

Is mutual masturbation okay?

Mutual masturbation is when couples stimulate themselves or each other without having intercourse. This is a sexual activity, and the Bible clearly says to avoid sexual activity like this until marriage.

God's design for sex is always between a husband and wife. If a male or female ever masturbates while thinking about someone other than their spouse, that is lust, which is a sin. That's why married people should not watch porn together, because it causes them to lust for others, which is the same as inviting other people into the marriage bed.

Is a wet dream a sin?

When a young man has a nocturnal emission, is that a sin? Many teen boys are really embarrassed by these and don't want anyone to know. They wonder, *Did I sin in my sleep?*

No, we can't control our dreams. And wet dreams are a normal body function when guys get a buildup of semen. (Side note: Guys who masturbate regularly will probably rarely, if at all, have wet dreams.)

We can't control dreams, but we can control what we fill our minds with. If we expose ourselves to sexual imagery, then our minds might dwell on some of that imagery.

Control your thoughts during the day and your nights will most likely follow. Wet dreams will still occur occasionally, and that's okay. As parents, we need to remember not to freak out about this. On the contrary, we should show extreme consideration for our son if we discover this embarrassing occurrence.

Why should I care if my looks or actions cause someone to lust? It's their own dirty mind, not my problem.

Believe it or not, some young people think like this. It's selfish and thoughtless.

But if you hear a question like this, rather than lecturing, ask questions. Maybe share Scriptures like these and then ask questions about the verses:

> Therefore let us stop passing judgment on one another. Instead, make up your mind not to put any stumbling block or obstacle in the way of a brother or sister.
>
> Romans 14:13 NIV

Ask:

- What does the verse say we shouldn't do?
- What is a stumbling block?
- What are some of the ways young men stumble today?
- How can you avoid causing them to stumble?

> Let us therefore make every effort to do what leads to peace and mutual edification.
>
> Romans 14:19 NIV

Ask:

- What are we to make every effort to do?
- What actions can we take that lead to peace and mutual edification?
- If someone has a dirty mind, what can we do to help edify them?

Is cohabitation okay?

This is a common question. I think it gets answered when we truly seek to understand God's plan for sex and marriage. In other words, if we are having frequent conversations with our kids about God's plan for sex (chapter 4), how far we can go (chapter 5), and fleeing (chapter 8), then this question will answer itself. But many young people today haven't been educated with the truth; instead, they've just been listening to the world's lies.

The world says, "You should test drive a car before you buy it. Couples should try living together to see if they are compatible."

The truth is, if a man and a woman wait until marriage for sex, then seek to humbly serve each other (Ephesians 5), sex and marriage are going to be amazing. Compatibility is for self-seeking individuals.

If two people move in together before marriage, the temptation will be to enjoy all the benefits of marriage without the commitment of marriage. This isn't God's plan and usually leads to pain and regret. In fact, couples who live together before marriage have a higher rate of divorce than couples who don't cohabitate before marriage.[3] Even more sobering, studies show that children of cohabiting couples are more likely to experience emotional problems, alcoholism, and drug abuse.[4] No one seems to know why, although experts speculate it might be because of the uncertainty of the relationship. In other words, the kids don't feel confident that Mom and Dad are really going to stick together. This has damaging effects.

Marriage vows often include the phrase "For better or worse." In other words, two people realize that there will be struggles when they are getting into a relationship. Conflict is a reality. Relationships take work, and hard work pays off. When two people enter a relationship with an attitude of "Let's try this, and we'll bail if it's difficult," the relationship is destined for failure. It's not a matter of *if* the relationship will fail . . . it's just a matter of *when*.

The "test drive" theory doesn't hold true. When Dad commits to Mom in marriage, it's better for their relationship and it's better for the kids.

How do I break out of an unhealthy cycle of sexual activity?

This is one of those questions parents should really celebrate.

Parents could look at a question like this as the glass being half empty. *My teen is sexually experienced.*

Don't make this mistake. The glass is half full. *My teen is looking for deliverance from a sexual past.*

Remember what we talked about in chapter 11 of this book. Whenever Jesus encountered someone with a blotted past, he didn't make them feel dirty; he made them feel forgiven and accepted. We should follow his example. When our teenagers mess up, we need to do everything we can to help them *not* feel like perverts.

But we can also help them break this unhealthy cycle.

If our teens want to break free of temptation, first determine if it's an addiction or just a habit of bad choices. If it's an addiction to porn, for example, you might need to bring them to counseling. An addiction is an addiction. (See chapter 9 for more about helping our kids break free of porn.)

But if your son or daughter has made a habit of sleeping with his or her girlfriend or boyfriend, then you can help them "flee" this kind of temptation. Let them know that they aren't alone, and in fact, most people endure this kind of temptation. But God is faithful to provide a way of escape (1 Corinthians 10:13).

I find that kids often don't think about the actions that lead to bad choices. Help them understand that most choices began five choices ago. If they keep having sex with their boyfriend or girlfriend, my guess is it's not at school in algebra class. It's probably after school, at someone's house, or in another private place.

Ask your daughter:

- Where are the places you are the most tempted?
- How can you avoid these places?
- Who is someone who can keep you accountable?

Sometimes our teens will be struggling with masturbation and they might see it as an addiction. If it is a porn addiction, then you might need to seek counseling. But if the kid just masturbates frequently, occasionally looking at images, then we can help them learn to try to flee this temptation. Help them by removing any of the easy access they have to images that are tempting. This might mean porn filters or cable blocks. It might mean even removing Mom's clothing catalogs with underwear ads. It's pretty difficult to remove everything, but do your best to help them flee.

And don't be surprised if your son continues to struggle with masturbation; it's a very hard habit to break. Your son is not dirty or perverted if he keeps doing it. He's struggling, as many of us do.

What if I don't get married? Does that mean I will never have sex, ever?!

The short answer: yes. Sex is for marriage. If you want to have sex, get married.

This isn't to say that remaining single is discouraged. In fact, the apostle Paul encouraged people to remain single if they were going to live a life of ministry. He says it like this:

> I say this as a concession, not as a command. But I wish everyone were single, just as I am. Yet each person has a special gift from God, of one kind or another.

> So I say to those who aren't married and to widows—it's better to stay unmarried, just as I am. But if they can't control themselves, they should go ahead and marry. It's better to marry than to burn with lust.
>
> 1 Corinthians 7:6–9

Paul was a missionary at heart. He traveled the world sharing the truth about Jesus, often getting arrested for standing up for truth. This was no life for a husband or father. That's why he wasn't afraid to give this personal little endorsement for staying single. He knew single people had more freedom to serve Jesus without any ties.

Yet at the same time, Paul knew the power of lust, so he made it clear: "If they can't control themselves, they should go ahead and marry. It's better to marry than to burn with lust."

Singleness has its benefits. But if you want sex and intimacy, then enjoy it the way God intended, in the relationship of marriage.

Is it wrong if I'm attracted to someone of the same sex?

This is just one of the many questions I've heard young people ask about homosexuality and same-sex attraction. Here are some other common questions:

> *"What's wrong with homosexual activity? If God made people with a certain desire, why would he forbid them from it?"*
>
> *"I don't like the opposite sex and I have feelings for the same sex. Does that mean I'm a homosexual?"*
>
> *"If I had a homosexual experience but am still attracted to the opposite sex, does that make me bisexual?"*

I confess, I was debating whether to even address this issue in this book. On one hand I know it's a common question that young people desperately need to hear truth about, but on the other hand, I know that the issue has grown so volatile that any answer on this issue divides people. So no matter what I write in these few pages, people are going to be looking for me to be one of two things: a *gay supporter*, or a *gay hater.*

If I had to choose one, I guess I'd have to be called a *gay supporter*, because I have gay friends and I love them. But I just happen to think that homosexual activity is a sin, just like looking at porn is a sin . . . as is lusting, cohabitating, and having premarital sex (not to mention gossiping, lying, and cheating on your taxes). Sadly, I have friends who are all of those things. Sadly, I am some of those things (in all honesty, I gossiped about someone last week). We all have something in common. We all need Jesus.

It's almost impossible to disagree with the homosexual lifestyle today without being labeled a hater. Questions about the issue are rarely asked without some emotion attached to them. Emotions are stirred because many young people who have experienced same-sex attraction have encountered teasing or bullying. Others might have kept these feelings to themselves but were afraid to ask questions. After all, the church has treated homosexuality as a uniquely terrible sin in the past. If you slept with your girlfriend or watched porn, that was one thing . . . but if you were gay? *Gasp!*

But the cultural climate has been changing rapidly in the last few years, and now homosexuality is almost completely accepted by the entertainment media community. If a celebrity were to speak out against homosexual behavior it would be career suicide. Movies, TV, and music frequently celebrate the homosexual lifestyle and are almost completely saturated with the message "How can something that feels so right be wrong?" This makes this issue increasingly difficult for parents because today's young people are absolutely immersed in entertainment media (peek at chapter 1 for a reminder of exactly how much).

Rappers Macklemore and Ryan Lewis spoke the minds of many of today's young people with their song "Same Love" in 2012. This song spoke out against bullying (a good thing to protest). It also called out right-wing conservatives, saying they were paraphrasing a book written thousands of years ago, a clear "dis" on the Bible's clarity and relevance. The world readily accepts this message. In fact, the 2014 Grammys featured the rap duo performing this song while Queen Latifah officiated a mass gay wedding on the stage in front of millions of viewers.

Today, if anyone is asked what they think about the homosexual lifestyle, they dare not speak their minds if they don't agree with it. They will be deemed intolerant or haters. As a result, many Christians are tiptoeing around the issue.

I don't tiptoe.

So I'll try to take the approach that Jesus took: *love* and *truth*. Jesus loved everyone, regardless of their sin; at the same time, he spoke the truth, even when it was very unpopular to do so.

Acting on Our Desires

Today the majority of young people think:

1. Homosexuals can't help but feel this way—they are "born this way."
2. We shouldn't judge them for feeling that way.
3. It's okay if they want to act on those desires.

Christians have been handling all three of these issues poorly. First, it's practically pointless to argue over number one, whether or not homosexuals are "born this way." This debate has never been settled either way, and frankly, it really doesn't need to be. Here's why: Desire isn't the issue—the issue is how we respond to our desires.

Think about it. We all know that some people are really prone to anger, some are prone to drinking, and some are prone to lust. Does that mean they should act out in these ways? Obviously not. I'm Irish and I have a really bad temper. Does that license me to go on tirades? Arguing about being "born this way" is really not relevant. The real issue is how I *act* on my desires.

Sadly, the church has been judging and mistreating homosexuals for years (number two above). This is ridiculous and against God's Word. First, we shouldn't judge any sinner; only God can judge. Most of the "correction" the Bible calls for is directed to believers in the church, and that is always supposed to be done in love. And as for condemning, even Jesus didn't come to condemn, but to save

(John 3:17). It's silly that the church would be hung up pointing the finger at homosexuals when the church is full of gossips, porn addicts, and greedy people. The church needs to show love and grace like Jesus did.

But that doesn't mean we should swing the pendulum and say, "Okay then, homosexual activity is *not* a sin."

The fact is, the Bible makes it clear about God's design for sexual activity. It's something we've been talking about in this entire book, so it should come as no surprise: one man, one woman in the context of marriage. In fact, the Bible even goes as far as to speak out against homosexual activity just as it speaks out against heterosexual sin. And not just in the Old Testament, but in the New Testament as well.

For example, in 1 Corinthians 6:9–11 (NIV), we read:

> Do you not know that wrongdoers will not inherit the kingdom of God? Do not be deceived: Neither the sexually immoral nor idolaters nor adulterers nor men who have sex with men nor thieves nor the greedy nor drunkards nor slanderers nor swindlers will inherit the kingdom of God. And that is what some of you were. But you were washed, you were sanctified, you were justified in the name of the Lord Jesus Christ and by the Spirit of our God.

In this passage, Paul is unmistakably condemning certain sins, with homosexuality being one of them—right along with greed and drunkenness—lest we think that one sinful lifestyle is worse (or better) than another. These are things Christians shouldn't be doing.

While some may want to see this passage as just another "clobber verse," it is best viewed as a passage of supreme hope! Instead of remaining in their sin, the Corinthians were washed, sanctified, and justified in the name of Jesus and by the power of God's Spirit! That's because God loves idolaters, adulterers, drunkards, thieves, slanderers, swindlers, and yes, homosexuals! I'm glad God's process of sanctification is at work in my life, because I'm really good at slandering people who make me mad. It's an area I've really needed to give to God, and he's slowly changing me.

In another of Paul's references to homosexuality, in 1 Timothy 1:9–11, he says:

> The law was not intended for people who do what is right. It is for people who are lawless and rebellious, who are ungodly and sinful, who consider nothing sacred and defile what is holy, who kill their father or mother or commit other murders. The law is for people who are sexually immoral, or who practice homosexuality, or are slave traders, liars, promise breakers, or who do anything else that contradicts the wholesome teaching that comes from the glorious Good News entrusted to me by our blessed God.

Here Paul lists those "who practice homosexuality" among the "lawless and rebellious." It is point-blank doctrine: Homosexuality is a lifestyle that's contradictory to the Gospel. But look what else Paul is doing. He's also clearly saying that God has reached out to the "lawless and rebellious" with his perfect law. Rather than condemn them, *God desires to redeem them*!

Romans chapter 1 paints it pretty plainly as well as Paul describes some of the shameful things mankind does, trading the truth about God for a lie:

> That is why God abandoned them to their shameful desires. Even the women turned against the natural way to have sex and instead indulged in sex with each other. And the men, instead of having normal sexual relations with women, burned with lust for each other. Men did shameful things with other men, and as a result of this sin, they suffered within themselves the penalty they deserved.
>
> vv. 26–27 NLT

The whole chapter is pretty clear that homosexual activity was not God's intent. It also details some other sins like greed, envy, and quarreling. (Funny, no one seems to be arguing that those actions are okay.)

While the Bible's mention of homosexuality seems completely straightforward, many argue that when the Bible uses the word *homosexual* it really means something else. Some argue that when the apostle Paul discusses homosexuality in 1 Corinthians 6:9 or 1 Timothy 1:10, what he was *really* denouncing was pederasty, the sexual abuse of boys by men, which was sometimes practiced by Roman and Greek citizens.

I have just one question: *Then why didn't Paul just say that?* You see, the apostle Paul was a man of profound specifics, who at times would even invent words to get his point across, like the concept of "justification" (Romans 4 and 5). Am I to believe that he simply began to use terms that were generic or vague or *even wrong* when talking about such important issues?

If Paul wanted to address adult-to-child sin, he would have done that. He didn't. The reason he didn't speak of pederasty was because he was referring to homosexuality.

But don't forget that these passages are all in the context of God's grace. All the passages above clearly communicate God's love for us and our need for his forgiveness. All of us need this love and grace.

How to Answer

So how do we answer our kids if they ask us about this issue?

1. Understand where they're coming from

Remember to ask a lot of questions. If your kids ask, "Dad, is it wrong to be gay?" Say to them, "That's a good question. Tell me more about the context of this question." Gather as much information as possible so you can be sensitive to their feelings. Ask them, "What do you think?" Remember, this is a very emotional issue for many.

2. Share Jesus' love for "sinners like me"

One of the biggest reasons the world dislikes Christians is because some Christians have come across as hateful and judgmental. Christ was neither of these things. In fact, Jesus claimed countless times that he came to save sinners. Help your kids understand that we are all sinners, and we need Jesus just like every sinner needs Jesus.

3. Share God's amazing plan for sex and marriage

Don't jump straight to a passage listing homosexuals among the immoral. Tell them God's story of how he created a husband and wife and told them to enjoy sex together. Share with them God's design for sex (chapter 4). Help them understand God's plan and what happens when people go outside of God's plan. Remember that many young people today don't see the Bible as an authority. So be prepared to discuss it beyond just "Because the Bible says so."

4. Help them understand that all sexual sin is outside of God's plan

Talk about homosexuality in the context of other sexual sins. Start by asking about other sexual sins. If a teenage boy really wants to sleep with his girlfriend, is it okay? Why not? If it feels right, how could it be wrong? If a man really wants to look at porn, can he? Why not? But he loves looking at naked women, how could that be wrong? What if they are under-aged women? Couldn't it be argued that he was born with these desires?

So should we follow every desire we have? The world loves to tell us that we should follow our every desire, but the truth is, sometimes our desires are sinful. We need to learn to follow God, not our own desires (Galatians 5:16–17).

5. Teach them the importance of resisting temptations

We need to teach our kids that if they are struggling with desires to engage in homosexual activity, God can help them resist that temptation (1 Corinthians 10:13), just like those who are struggling with lust, porn, or any heterosexual sin. Yes, most of us are in the same boat, struggling with temptations, and we need Jesus badly. (Read more about fleeing sexual sin in chapter 8 of this book.)

Our world is confused by this messy issue. Sadly, homosexuals have been bullied. This is a tragedy. It should have never happened. Sadly, homosexuals have been judged and singled out. This has made it very difficult for those struggling with same-sex attraction.

As Christians, we need to love homosexuals just like we need to love a porn addict or the heterosexual couple that lives next door that has been cohabitating for six years but still isn't married. When we model this kind of love to others, our kids will be attracted to Christ's love in us. In the same way, if our kids struggle with feelings of same-sex attraction, we need to treat them with the same love and grace that we'd treat our kids struggling with porn or any other sexual temptation.

Pray through this whole process. Pray specifically that God will help you live out these principles and answer these questions in love and truth. And remember, our love will point to truth loudly.

A Parent Question:

This last question is a common "tough question" I've heard from parents. I think it's worth addressing.

Should we tell our kids about our mistakes?

I have a friend who asked me this: "Our daughter was born seven months after our wedding date. It's only a matter of time before she does the math and asks us why. When should we tell her that we had premarital sex?"

Great question. And the short answer is, *whenever she asks.*

I don't think you need to bring it up to your five-year-old. She won't understand. And I don't think you need to bring it up to your thirteen-year-old out of the blue. My guess is, if you are engaging in frequent conversations about sex and dating, it will come up naturally at some point. When it does, share the truth.

There is some debate out there as to whether we should share our bad decisions with our kids. I've read articles urging parents to keep quiet because it gives our kids permission to act out.

I think stories about past mistakes can be good or bad, depending on context and approach. If a parent is joking or bragging about all the stupid things they did, then yes, don't be surprised if these behaviors are imitated. After all, *"Dad did it!"*

But I've seen countless examples of a dad or mom sharing the hurt of past mistakes, with tears and sincerity, and it's helped his or her children realize they don't want to experience that kind of hurt.

Today's young people are being inundated with messages of "sex is recreational" and "do it" with no mention of consequences. I think it's powerful when a parent shares stories of choices and their consequences.

Never be afraid to share the truth.

When we're vulnerable and honest, it can help set the stage for our kids to be vulnerable and honest. And isn't that what we want?

Are you creating a climate of continual conversations about sex?

Are you becoming your kids' go-to person about sex?

What Now?

So what now?

Near the beginning of this book I shared a study from the journal *Pediatrics* entitled, "Beyond the 'Big Talk,'" encouraging parents to consider having repeated discussions with their children about many aspects of sex instead of just one "big talk."

In study after study we've seen the same thing, and the Bible would agree. In fact, in Deuteronomy chapter 6, Moses told God's people:

> And you must commit yourselves wholeheartedly to these commands that I am giving you today. Repeat them again and again to your children. Talk about them when you are at home and when you are on the road, when you are going to bed and when you are getting up.
>
> Deuteronomy 6:6–7

The mandate is clear. Keep having these conversations. It's our calling as parents. We have an awesome opportunity to create a comfortable climate for continual conversations, even about tough issues like sex and intimacy.

Yes, this can be a little scary. Especially when those conversations become explicit.

I think it's worth repeating that the *Pediatrics* study not only concluded, "The more parents talked with their children, the closer their relationships," but the relationship between parent and child really benefitted "when the discussions moved beyond 'safe' or impersonal subjects such as puberty, reproduction and sexually transmitted diseases to more private topics such as masturbation and how sex feels."[1]

Perhaps "explicit" isn't so bad when it's true.

Are you ready for these conversations?

What is your first step?

Notes

Start Here: Unanswered Questions

1. Laura Kann, PhD, Steve Kinchen, Shari L. Shanklin, MPH, et al., "Youth Risk Behavior Surveillance—United States," *MMWR* 63, no. 4(2014): 112, www.cdc.gov/mmwr/pdf/ss/ss6304.pdf.
2. Pam Stenzel, *HomeWord Daily* radio show with Dr. Jim Burns, March 20, 2007.
3. "Nationally Representative CDC Study Finds 1 in 4 Teenage Girls Has a Sexually Transmitted Disease," Centers for Disease Control and Prevention, March 10, 2008, www.cdc.gov/stdconference/2008/press/release-11march2008.htm.
4. "HPV and Cancer," National Cancer Institute at the National Institutes of Health, March 15, 2012, www.cancer.gov/cancertopics/factsheet/Risk/HPV.
5. "Chlamydia—CDC Fact Sheet," Centers for Disease Control and Prevention, January 2013, www.cdc.gov/Std/chlamydia/STDFact-Chlamydia.htm.

Chapter 1: The Loud Voices

1. Wiz Khalifa, "No Sleep" from *Rolling Papers*, written by Cameron Thomaz and Benjamin Levin, Atlantic Records and Rostrum Records, 2011.
2. Gilbert Cruz, Amanda Dobbins, Jesse David Fox, Margaret Lyons, Lindsey Weber, and Nate Jones, "100 Pop-Culture Things That Make You a Millennial," *Vulture,* September 24, 2013, www.vulture.com/2013/09/100-pop-culture-things-that-make-you-millennial.html#photo=20x00068.
3. *McAfee Digital Deception Study 2013: Exploring the Online Disconnect between Parents & Pre-teens, Teens and Young Adults*, June 2013, www.mcafee.com/us/resources/reports/rp-digital-deception-survey.pdf, 18.
4. Ibid., 16.

5. Victoria J. Rideout, MA, Ulla G. Foehr, PhD, and Donald F. Roberts, PhD, *Generation M²: Media in the Lives of 8- to 18-Year-Olds*, The Henry J. Kaiser Family Foundation, January 2010, http://kaiserfamilyfoundation.files.wordpress.com/2013/04/8010.pdf.

6. "Dirty song lyrics can prompt early teen sex," NBCnews.com, August 7, 2006, www.nbcnews.com/id/14227775/ns/health-sexual_health/t/dirty-song-lyrics-can-prompt-early-teen-sex/#.UksbarwmYhc.

7. Don Reisinger, "91 percent of kids are gamers, research says," CNET, October 11, 2011, www.cnet.com/news/91-percent-of-kids-are-gamers-research-says.

8. Rideout, Foehr, and Roberts.

9. "Nielsen Releases Quarterly Report on Cross-Platform Media Audience Behavior," Nielsen.com, June 15, 2011, www.nielsen.com/us/en/press-room/2011/q1-cross-platform-report.html.

10. "Entertainment Weekly's Top 100 TV Shows," *Your TV Tour Guide*, July 2, 2013, http://tvtourguide.blogspot.com/2013/07/entertainment-weeklys-top-100-tv-shows.html.

11. Hollie McKay, "FCC proposing to allow more sex and profanity during kids' television viewing hours," FoxNews.com, May 21, 2013, www.foxnews.com/entertainment/2013/05/21/fcc-proposing-to-allow-more-sex-and-profanity-during-kids-television-viewing.

12. Rebecca Hagelin, "Study shows teens imitate risky sex of films, TV," *The Washington Times,* August 12, 2012, www.washingtontimes.com/news/2012/aug/12/hagelin-study-shows-teens-imitate-risky-sex-of-fil/#ixzz2gUzHLlc0.

13. Ibid.

14. "Pornography Statistics," XXXchurch, www.xxxchurch.com/extras/pornographystatistics.html.

15. "Pornography Statistics: Annual Report 2014," Covenant Eyes, www.covenanteyes.com/pornstats.

16. Ibid.

17. "Teen Olympia Nelson takes stand against sexualised selfie photos," ABC News Australia, September 23, 2013, www.abc.net.au/news/2013–09–23/australian-story-olympia-nelson-takes-stand-on-sexualised-selfie/4973912.

18. Olympia Nelson, "Dark undercurrents of teenage girls' selfies," *The Age*, July 11, 2013, www.theage.com.au/comment/dark-undercurrents-of-teenage-girls-selfies-20130710-2pqbl.html.

19. Simon Khalaf , "Flurry Five-Year Report: It's an App World. The Web Just Lives in It," Flurry, April 3, 2013, www.flurry.com/bid/95723/Flurry-Five-Year-Report-It-s-an-App-World-The-Web-Just-Lives-in-It#.U-pkG1M1Cuk.

20. Nancy Jo Sales, "Friends Without Benefits," *Vanity Fair*, September 26, 2013, www.vanityfair.com/culture/2013/09/social-media-Internet-porn-teenage-girls.

21. Ibid.

Chapter 2: The Quiet Voices

1. Anne Marie Miller, "3 Things You Don't Know About Your Children and Sex," Church Leaders, www.churchleaders.com/youth/youth-leaders-articles/169715-anne-marie-miller-things-you-know-about-your-children-and-sex.html.

2. "Pornography Statistics: Annual Report 2014," Covenant Eyes, www.covenant eyes.com/pornstats.

3. Mark Oestreicher, "What's the Difference Between Teaching Middle Schoolers and High Schoolers About Dating and Sexuality?" *whyismarko*, February 6, 2012, http://whyismarko.com/whats-the-difference-between-teaching-middle-schoolers-and-high-schoolers-about-dating-and-sexuality.

4. Ibid.

5. Stephanie Desmon, "Study: 1 in 4 teen girls has an STD," *Boston Globe*, March 12, 2008, www.boston.com/news/health/articles/2008/03/12/study_1_in_4_teen_girls_has_an_std.

6. Kathleen Doheny, "Many Teen Girls Mistakenly Think HPV Vaccines Cut Risk for All STDs," *U.S. News and World Report*, January 5, 2012, http://health.usnews.com/health-news/family-health/cancer/articles/2012/01/05/many-teen-girls-mistakenly-think-hpv-vaccines-cut-risk-for-all-stds.

7. Andrew Stern, "Parents Urged to Go Beyond 'Big Talk' About Sex," Reuters, March 3, 2008, www.reuters.com/article/2008/03/03/us-sex-adolescents-parents-idUSN2920679220080303.

Chapter 3: Opening the Doorways of Communication

1. Martin Daubney, "Experiment that convinced me online porn is the most pernicious threat facing children today," *Mail Online*, September 25, 2013, www.dailymail.co.uk/femail/article-2432591/Porn-pernicious-threat-facing-children-today-By-ex-lads-mag-editor-MARTIN-DAUBNEY.html.

2. Zoe Ruderman, "The Scary New Butt Beauty Trend," *Cosmopolitan*, August 3, 2011, http://www.cosmopolitan.com/health-fitness/advice/a3634/anal-bleaching-trend.

3. "Injury Prevention & Control: Motor Vehicle Safety—Teen Drivers: Fact Sheet," Centers for Disease Control and Prevention, October 7, 2014, cdc.gov/motorvehiclesafety/teen_drivers/teendrivers_factsheet.html.

Chapter 4: The Most Enjoyable Sex

1. Kann, Kinchen, Shanklin, et al.

2. G. Martinez, C. E. Copen, and J. C. Abma, *Teenagers in the United States: Sexual Activity, Contraceptive Use, and Childbearing, 2006–2010 National Survey of Family Growth*. National Center for Health Statistics 23, no. 31 (2011): 11, 26, www.cdc.gov/nchs/data/series/sr_23/sr23_031.pdf.

3. Maia Szalavitz, "How Oxytocin Makes Men (Almost) Monogamous," *Time*, November 27, 2013, http://healthland.time.com/2013/11/27/how-oxytocin-makes-men-almost-monogamous.

4. Ross Douthat, "Why Monogamy Matters," *The New York Times*, March 6, 2011, www.nytimes.com/2011/03/07/opinion/07douthat.html?_r=0.

5. E. O. Laumann, J. H. Gagnon, R. T. Michael, and S. Michaels, *The Social Organization of Sexuality: Sexual Practices in the United States*, (Chicago: The University of Chicago Press, 1994).

6. Ibid., 115.

7. Ibid.

8. R. J. Levin and A. Levin, "Sexual Pleasure: The Surprising Preferences of 100,000 Women," *Redbook,* September 1975, 51–58.

9. David G. Blanchflower and Andrew J. Oswald, *Money, Sex, and Happiness: An Empirical Study* (National Bureau of Economic Research Working Paper No. 10499, May 2004), cited in David R. Francis, "Monogamy Is Good—And Good For You," *The Christian Science Monitor,* December 5, 2005, www.csmonitor.com/2005/1205/p15s01-cogn.html.

10. Mark D. White, PhD, "On Monogamy, Happiness, and Adultery," *Psychology Today*, March 12, 2011, www.psychologytoday.com/blog/maybe-its-just-me/201103/monogamy-happiness-and-adultery.

11. "HPV and Cancer," National Cancer Institute at the National Institutes of Health, www.cancer.gov/cancertopics/factsheet/Risk/HPV.

12. "Abortion Facts," National Abortion Federation, www.prochoice.org/about_abortion/facts/women_who.html.

Chapter 6: Your Daughter

1. Vivian Diller, PhD, "Sex and the Single Teen: Internet Porn and Body Image," *Huffington Post*, August 20, 2012, www.huffingtonpost.com/vivian-diller-phd/Internet-porn-body-image_b_1777026.html.

2. "Report of the APA Task Force on the Sexualization of Girls: Executive Summary," American Psychological Association, 2007, www.apa.org/pi/wpo/sexualization.html.

3. Matt Thomas, "Going Gaga," *fab* magazine, http://ladygaga.wikia.com/wiki/Fab_%28magazine%29.

4. Rideout, Foehr, and Roberts.

5. Randy Dotinga, "Dad's Advice Could Be Key to Teens' Sexual Activity," *U.S. News and World Report*, October 18, 2012, http://health.usnews.com/health-news/news/articles/2012/10/18/dads-advice-could-be-key-to-teens-sexual-activity.

Chapter 7: Your Son

1. Rideout, Foehr, and Roberts.

2. "U.S. Teens Use Game Consoles More for Internet than Gaming," eMarketer, February 28, 2014, www.emarketer.com/Article/US-Teens-Use-Game-Consoles-More-Internet-than-Gaming/1010647/3.

3. David Segal, "Does Porn Hurt Children?" *The New York Times*, March 28, 2014, www.nytimes.com/2014/03/29/sunday-review/does-porn-hurt-children.html?_r=1.

4. Rebecca Hagelin, "Study shows teens imitate risky sex of films, TV," *The Washington Times*, August 12, 2012, www.washingtontimes.com/news/2012/aug/12/hagelin-study-shows-teens-imitate-risky-sex-of-fil/#ixzz2gUzHLlc0.

5. Mark Matlock, Twitter post, May 13, 2014, 6:54 a.m., https://twitter.com/MarkMatlock/status/466214851275390976.

Chapter 8: Fleeing

1. "Infidelity Statistics," Statistic Brain, January 1, 2014, www.statisticbrain.com/infidelity-statistics.

2. "Freshman women's binge drinking tied to sexual assault risk," *Science Blog*, December 8, 2011, http://scienceblog.com/50305/freshman-womens-binge-drinking-tied-to-sexual-assault-risk, citing Testa, M., & Hoffman, J. H. (January 2012). "Naturally occurring changes in women's drinking from high school to college and implications for sexual victimization," *Journal of Studies on Alcohol and Drugs,* 73(1), 26.

Chapter 9: The Lure of Porn

1. Sean McDowell, "The Hidden Price Tag of Porn," Church Leaders, www.churchleaders.com/pastors/pastor-articles/156270-the-hidden-price-tag-of-porn.html.

2. "Pornography Statistics: Annual Report 2014," Covenant Eyes, www.covenanteyes.com/pornstats.

3. "Children and Pornography," Center for Parent/Youth Understanding, www.digitalkidsinitiative.com/files/2014/08/Children_and_Pornography_Factsheet-Revised-August-2014.pdf

4. "Pornography Statistics," www.covenanteyes.com/pornstats.

5. Ibid.

6. Natalie Matthews, "See All the Ridiculously Hot, Nearly Naked Looks from Shakira and Rihanna's New Video," *Elle*, January 31, 2014, www.elle.com/news/culture/shakira-rihanna-cant-remember-forget-you-outfits-video.

7. Miller, "3 Things You Don't Know About Your Children and Sex."

8. Cecilia Kang, "Seeking Privacy, Teens Turn to Anonymous-Messaging Apps," *The Washington Post*, February 16, 2014, www.washingtonpost.com/business/technology/seeking-privacy-teens-turn-to-anonymous-messaging-apps/2014/02/16/1ffa583a-9362-11e3-b46a-5a3d0d2130da_story.html.

9. Penny Marshall, "Teenage Boys Watching Hours of Internet Pornography Every Week Are Treating Their Girlfriends Like Sex Objects," *Mail Online*, March 8, 2010, www.dailymail.co.uk/news/article-1255856/Teenage-boys-watching-hours-Internet-pornography-week-treating-girlfriends-like-sex-objects.html.

10. "Children, Adolescents, and the Media," *Pediatrics* 132, no. 5 (November 1, 2013): 958–961, http://pediatrics.aappublications.org/content/132/5/958.full.

11. "Internet Porn Making Men Bad in Bed," *International Business Times*, October 24, 2011, www.ibtimes.co.uk/Internet-porn-making-men-bad-in-bed-porn-xxx-pornography-sex-sexual-intercourse-cam2cam-erectile-dys-236295.

12. M. Robinson and G. Wilson, "Cupid's Poisoned Arrow: Porn-Induced Sexual Dysfunction Growing Problem," *Psychology Today,* July 11, 2011.

13. Ibid.

Chapter 10: Providing Answers About Masturbation

1. Laumann, Gagnon, Michael, and Michaels, *The Social Organization of Sexuality: Sexual Practices in the United States.*

2. "Love Yourself!" *Seventeen*, www.seventeen.com/health/tips/love-yourself.

3. Alan Mozes, "Study Tracks Masturbation Trends Among U.S. Teens," *U.S. News and World Report*, August 1, 2011, http://health.usnews.com/health-news/

family-health/womens-health/articles/2011/08/01/study-tracks-masturbation-trends-among-us-teens.

4. "Millennials in Adulthood," PewResearch, March 7, 2014, www.pewsocialtrends.org/2014/03/07/millennials-in-adulthood.

5. Stern, "Parents Urged to Go Beyond 'Big Talk' About Sex."

6. Bonnie Rochman, "Who Are Teens' Sexual Role Models? Turns Out, It's Their Parents," *Time*, July 18, 2011, http://healthland.time.com/2011/07/18/surprise-teens-consider-parents-their-sexual-role-models.

7. Jordan Monge, "The Real Problem With Female Masturbation," *Christianity Today*, April 2014, www.christianitytoday.com/women/2014/april/real-problem-with-female-masturbation.html.

8. Martinez, Copen, and Abma, "Teenagers in the United States: Sexual Activity, Contraceptive Use, and Childbearing."

9. John Piper, "ANTHEM: Strategies for Fighting Lust," Desiring God, November 5, 2001, www.desiringgod.org/articles/anthem-strategies-for-fighting-lust.

Chapter 11: Surviving a Blotted Past

1. Kann, Kinchen, Shanklin, et al, "Youth Risk Behavior Surveillance —United States, 2013."

2. "Child Sexual Abuse Statistics," The National Center for Victims of Crime, www.victimsofcrime.org/media/reporting-on-child-sexual-abuse/child-sexual-abuse-statistics.

3. Dean G. Kilpatrick, Benjamin E. Saunders, and Daniel W. Smith, *Youth Victimization: Prevalence and Implications* (Washington, D.C.: U.S. Department of Justice, 2003), 5.

Chapter 12: Tough Questions

1. Randye Hoder, "Study Finds Most Teens Sext Before They're 18," *Time*, July 3, 2014, http://time.com/2948467/chances-are-your-teen-is-sexting.

2. Dr. Sanjay Gupta, "Have you had the 'sext' talk with your kids?" CNN Health, June 30, 2014, http://thechart.blogs.cnn.com/2014/06/30/have-you-had-the-sext-talk-with-your-kids.

3. Casey E. Copen, PhD; Kimberly Daniels, PhD; Jonathan Vespa, PhD; and William D. Mosher, PhD, "First Marriages in the United States: Data From the 2006–2010 National Survey of Family Growth," *National Health Statistics Reports*, no. 49, March 22, 2012, 2, www.cdc.gov/nchs/data/nhsr/nhsr049.pdf.

4. Sharon Jayson, "Living Together: No Big Deal?" *USA Today*, March 26, 2011, http://usatoday30.usatoday.com/printedition/life/20080609/d_worldcohab09.art.htm.

What Now?

1. Stern, "Parents Urged to Go Beyond 'Big Talk' About Sex."

Jonathan McKee is an expert on youth culture and the author of more than a dozen books, including *Get Your Teenager Talking, Sex Matters, The Zombie Apocalypse Survival Guide for Teenagers,* and *The Guy's Guide to God, Girls, and the Phone in Your Pocket.* He has twenty years of youth-ministry experience and speaks to parents and leaders worldwide. He also writes about parenting and youth culture while providing free resources at TheSource4Parents.com. Jonathan, his wife, Lori, and their three kids live in California.

For more information, go to JonathanMcKeeWrites.com and follow Jonathan on Twitter.com/InJonathansHead.

More From Jonathan McKee

Jonathan writes about parenting and provides free resources at TheSource4Parents.com.

The Teen Companion to *More Than Just the Talk*

Written directly to young people, *Sex Matters* gives teens the whole truth about sex and God's design for it. With straight talk and clear answers, McKee reveals that society hasn't been telling the whole truth about sex. Beyond the possibility of pregnancy and STDs, there are emotional and relational consequences to engaging in sex at the wrong time. *Sex Matters* celebrates sex in the context of marriage, but also highlights the dangers of misusing sex outside this context.

Sex Matters

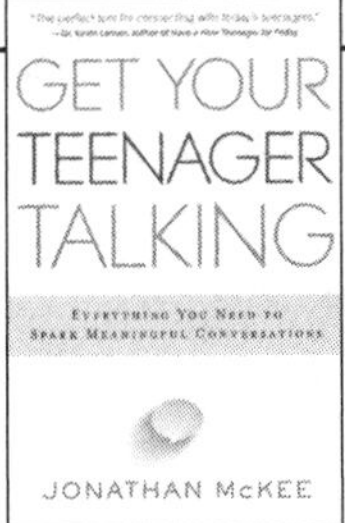

In this book, Jonathan McKee shares 180 creative discussion starters to help you get your teen to open up about issues that matter. You'll also find tips for interpreting their responses and follow-up questions. From lighthearted to more serious, these conversation springboards will encourage even the most reluctant teen to talk about friends, school, values, struggles, and much more.

Get Your Teenager Talking